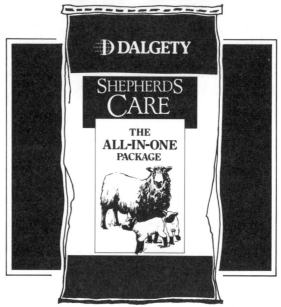
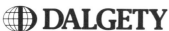
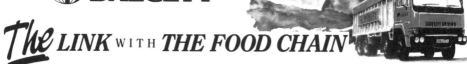

Planned Sheep Production

Planned Sheep Production

Second Edition

David Croston
and
Geoff Pollott

OXFORD

BLACKWELL SCIENTIFIC PUBLICATIONS

LONDON EDINBURGH BOSTON

MELBOURNE PARIS BERLIN VIENNA

© D. Croston & G.E. Pollott 1985, 1994

Blackwell Scientific Publications
Editorial Offices:
Osney Mead, Oxford OX2 0EL
25 John Street, London WC1N 2BL
23 Ainslie Place, Edinburgh EH3 6AJ
238 Main Street, Cambridge,
   Massachusetts, 02142, USA
54 University Street, Carlton,
   Victoria 3053, Australia

Other Editorial Offices:
Librairie Arnette SA
1, rue de Lille
75007 Paris
France

Blackwell Wissenschafts-Verlag GmbH
Düsseldorfer Str. 38
D-10707 Berlin
Germany

Blackwell MZV
Feldgasse 13
A-1238 Wien
Austria

First Edition published by Collins
   Professional and Technical Books 1985
Second Edition published by Blackwell
   Scientific Publications 1994

Set by DP Photosetting, Aylesbury, Bucks
Printed and bound in Great Britain by
Hartnolls Ltd, Bodmin, Cornwall

DISTRIBUTORS

Marston Book Services Ltd
PO Box 87
Oxford OX2 0DT
(*Orders*: Tel: 0865 791155
         Fax: 0865 791927
         Telex: 837515)

USA
Blackwell Scientific Publications, Inc.
238 Main Street
Cambridge, MA 02142
(*Orders*: Tel: 800 759-6102
             617 876 7000)

Canada
Oxford University Press
70 Wynford Drive
Don Mills
Ontario M3C 1J9
(*Orders*: Tel: (416) 441-2941)

Australia
Blackwell Scientific Publications Pty Ltd
54 University Street
Carlton, Victoria 3053
(*Orders*: Tel: 03 347-5552)

British Library
Cataloguing in Publication Data
A Catalogue record for this book is available
from the British Library

ISBN 0–632–03576–5

Library of Congress
Cataloging in Publication Data
Croston, David.
   Planned sheep production/David Croston
   and Geoff Pollott.—2nd ed.
       p.   cm.
   Includes bibliographical references (p.   )
   and index.
   ISBN 0–632–03576–5
   1. Sheep.   2. Sheep—Great Britain.
   I. Pollott, Geoffrey.
II. Title.
SF375.C82   1993
636.3—dc20
                            93-27501
                               CIP

Contents

Preface to First Edition   vii

Preface to Second Edition   ix

1 A Planned Approach   **1**
Financial aspects of planning   3
Planning aids   6
Planning examples   9

Section 1: Aspects of Production   **17**

2 World Trade and Production   **19**
The world sheep population   19
Sheep products   23
Systems and environments   32

3 United Kingdom Production Statistics   **38**
EC sheep production   38
Production in the United Kingdom   46

Section 2: Resources   **53**

4 Animal Resources   **55**
Breeding ewes   55
Breeding rams   72
Lamb growth and carcase characteristics   77
Lamb marketing   83
The genetic improvement of animal resources   93

5 Feed Resources   **109**
Grass   109

Forage crops 124
Conserved forages 126
Concentrate feeds 127

6 Fixed Resources **129**
Land 131
Labour 132
Capital 133
Housing and equipment 136

7 Exploiting Resources **140**
Purebreeding 140
Self-contained pure and crossbreeding 141
Crossbreeding 143

Section 3: Production Systems **149**

8 Hill Sheep Production **151**
Resources 153
Increasing output from hill flocks 156
Resource management 162

9 Upland Sheep Production **164**
Products 166
Production systems 168

10 Lowland Sheep Production **175**
Products 176
Production systems 180

References 197

Index 203

Preface to First Edition

In most countries of the world sheep production is carried out as a secondary farm enterprise and as such does not always receive the inputs required to optimize output. One of the aims of this book is to show how careful planning of the sheep enterprise, whatever its status on the farm, can result in a more efficient use of resources. We have used the British sheep industry as our main source of material for obvious reasons, but have also used examples from other countries to demonstrate how certain principles have a wide application.

A book such as this cannot deal solely with the technical aspects of sheep production. Every farm enterprise exists in a particular economic and political situation which necessarily dictates some of the constraints on the enterprise. These 'extra-farm factors' must be taken into account when plans are drawn up, and attention to possible changes in the wider aspects of sheep production is essential.

We have, therefore, set out to describe the position of sheep in the world and outline some of the mechanisms of the trade in sheep products. In order that later points concerning the British sheep industry are fully understood, aspects of the European Community (EC) and in particular the Common Agricultural Policy (CAP) for sheepmeat are described. This then leads to a full consideration of the important resources available to producers including the stock themselves, feed resources and finally fixed resources. Systems of sheep production in Britain are examined in some detail to highlight the more important aspects of planning which have been discussed in earlier sections.

During the writing of this book we have been very conscious of the fact that its content reflects our own experience and interests. Certain aspects of sheep production such as nutrition, sheep breeding, sheep health and flock management each warrant a complete book on their own. We have discussed these subjects where appropriate but for a more complete consideration of them more detailed texts than our own should be consulted.

Finally we are indebted to many people who have helped us with the writing of this book. Our thanks are due to our employers, the Meat and Livestock Commission (MLC), for permission both to write the book in the first place and to draw extensively on their data and publications. Needless to say, any opinions expressed in this book are entirely our own. We are also greatly indebted to Mr J. L. Read, Head of MLC's Sheep Improvement Services, for his constant help and encouragement not only during the writing of this book but also during our years at the Commission. We would also like to thank Brian Kilkenny for his help and encouragement in setting up the book in the first place.

Preface to Second Edition

Positive comments from various users of our First Edition and their exhortations to review and update the book have given us the encouragement to prepare this Second Edition. Great political changes have taken place in various parts of the world since the first edition and the CAP has undergone a major overhaul. The breakup of the USSR is of course very significant for world sheep production and consumption, given its major role in both fields. However no statistical data is yet available from the now independent countries that made up the USSR and therefore we have been obliged to treat them collectively as the 'former USSR'. Despite all these changes the principles we advocate still hold good and our efforts have therefore focused on additions and updates to reflect these important changes.

In this ever-changing environment, for any enterprise to survive and hopefully thrive, it is necessary to keep abreast of all the latest techniques and developments in order to plan for the future. With this Second Edition we hope that by updating the evidence and including the new developments we will provide a framework to enable the planned production of sheep to be as profitable and successful an enterprise as economic conditions allow.

David Croston
Geoff Pollott

1 A Planned Approach

Profitable sheep production will be achieved provided that the chosen system of production optimizes resource use and is operated as efficiently and economically as possible. Systematic planning of the enterprise enables some form of production targets to be set and, through monitoring, can provide a realistic evaluation of the consequences of falling short of the set targets. Planning serves as a guide in the decision making process, whether for a new enterprise plan or the modification of an existing one (Fig. 1.1). Either way, data is required to feed the decision making process. Ideas and information, from whatever sources they are available, need to be assimilated

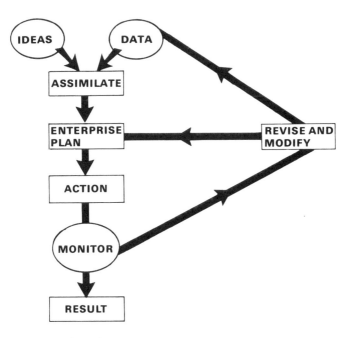

Fig. 1.1 Planning flowchart

before incorporation into an enterprise plan. Its implementation will generate data and information which, through the monitoring process, can be used if necessary to revise and modify the original enterprise plan and source data. The results of this first action may be less than perfect but, through monitoring and revision of the key aspects, plans can continually be improved.

Prospective sheep producers must answer two questions in order to initiate their production plans:

(1) What product should I aim for?
(2) On what scale should the product be produced?

Only then can decisions be made on how best to invest the available resources of capital and land, the number of staff required and how the choice of system will integrate with other enterprises on the farm.

In practice, choice is limited by the physical factors of the land, soil type and climate, the equipment and labour available and the general economy at the time. Existing producers will have arrived at a plan of some kind but this may not necessarily have been clearly defined. For example, recent changes in the EC agricultural policy have forced British sheep producers to reassess their farming enterprises and review their plans. If the market demand for the product is to be met, producers must be aware of any possible flexibility within their own system which will allow them to move with the times. Important planning decisions are generally long term, however, and are not normally able to undergo sudden changes. In fact frequent alterations to any plans are disruptive and expensive, and should be avoided wherever possible.

Whatever objective is foremost in the planner's mind, other motives may be important to the producer. The latter's choice of breed or system of production, for example, may be influenced by his own particular preferences and these may be considered counterproductive by the planner. However, such indulgences can be economically justified up to a point if they minimize stress and therefore make success more likely.

Experience with recorded flocks in Britain during a period of expansion in the sheep industry shows that success is not achieved simply by stringing all the available technical knowledge together in a single package. There is no 'blueprint for success' and no universal answer because, with the diversity of type, products and locations, no two sheep farms are the same. However, success is seldom the result of chance and it is possible to define certain principles which will help to generate the right plan for a particular set of circumstances. In the final analysis, success depends on the individual's expertise in dealing with all the critical areas of the enterprise.

A basic requirement of planning is access to the wide range of physical and financial data which is needed to formulate plans for any sheep enterprise. A number of national recording schemes were surveyed in 1986 (Pollott, Flamant, Jankowski, Tchakerian & Trodahl, 1987). These are organized to provide participants with the data necessary to monitor their own flock performance and, by the aggregation of individual results, to provide valuable targets and measurements of performance for wider industry use. In Britain the Meat and Livestock Commission (MLC) operates such a scheme, called Flockplan, which provides a wealth of valuable physical and financial data at individual farm, regional and national levels. In countries where recording schemes do not exist, data produced by state research institutes or large individual farms become the main source of reference material. Planning without access to figures of this kind is virtually impossible.

Financial aspects of planning

One accepted method of comparing enterprises on the farm makes use of the 'gross margin' concept, gross margin being defined as the gross output of the flock minus the variable costs of production. A new sheep enterprise under consideration, or an existing one, can be assessed in this manner. The financial framework, which can be expressed in terms of individual animal, flock or unit area, is as shown in the table at the top of page 4.

A typical gross margin calculation for a lowland spring lambing flock selling most of the lambs off grass in the summer is presented in Table 1.1. Flock replacement cost is the annual cost of maintaining the breeding stock. The number of replacements required annually and their purchase price in relation to the price received for culled breeding stock determines this cost. Figures are presented per ewe mated, which is the basis widely adopted in Britain. In other countries this may not be appropriate. For example, in Norway production statistics and costs are expressed per winter-fed ewe.

The gross margin of a single enterprise must not be looked at in isolation. Yearly fluctuations in annual performance are sometimes

GROSS OUTPUT	Total receipts from sheep products, e.g. lamb sales, wool
minus VARIABLE COSTS	E.g. purchased and home grown feeds.
equals GROSS MARGIN	
minus FIXED COSTS	Not generally assigned to a single enterprise.
equals NET PROFIT	Normally expressed for the whole farm.

Table 1.1 Example gross margin for lowland ewe flock.

	£ per ewe
Output	
Lamb sales	64.98
Wool sales	2.26
Ewe premium (subsidy)	10.32
Gross returns	77.56
Less flock replacement cost	6.51
Output	71.05
Variable costs	
Ewe concentrates	8.82
Lamb concentrates	12.69
Purchased forage	0.82
Fertilizer	3.27
Other forage costs	2.41
Vet and medicine	3.88
Miscellaneous and transport	3.33
Total variable costs	35.22
Gross margin (output minus variable costs)	35.83

forgotten, and any enterprise should be considered over a two or three year period in order to obtain a true picture of the levels of physical and financial performance. Aggregate data from a number of similar enterprises recorded in the same year provides a more valuable yardstick against which to measure an existing enterprise or budget for a planned one.

Performance targets

Flockplan records highlight the tremendous variation in both physical and financial performance, and the range of results likely to be achieved. The data from flocks having the best levels of performance can be used as a target for other sheep enterprises of the same type. MLC uses the concept of the 'top third' for this purpose.

If results are ranked on a given criterion, e.g. gross margin per hectare, then the average results for the best third of flocks become the top third. A comparison of top third financial results for lowland spring lambing flocks against the average of all flocks emphasizes the wide variation (Table 1.2). A similar comparison of some of the more important physical characters makes the same point (Table 1.3).

The top third flocks achieve higher output, mainly through rearing more lambs per ewe, and have a lower level of costs. They manage land resources considerably better and therefore achieve higher stocking rates. The components of success in these flocks can be summarized as:

- Higher stocking rates
- More lambs reared
- Higher lamb value
- Lower costs of production
- Lower replacement costs

Over a wide range of systems of production in Britain, these few components of success are paramount. The contribution that each makes to the top third superiority in gross margin per hectare may be estimated by reference to Table 1.4.

The simple concept of the top third is found to be most useful in the identification of key areas of flock profitability and valuable for advising commercial producers of important factors warranting close attention. The need for this type of yardstick will apply in any situation and a great number of sheep producers will be able to compare their own performance against such data.

In many cases outside technical advice is required, and anyone

Table 1.2 Financial results for lowland spring lambing flocks, 1991. (Source: MLC, 1992a)

	(£ per ewe)	
	Average	Top third
Output		
Lamb sales	50.59	56.28
Wool sales	2.19	2.21
Ewe premium	9.92	10.38
Gross returns	62.70	68.87
Less flock replacement cost	7.30	6.49
Output	55.40	62.38
Variable costs		
Ewe concentrates	7.53	7.10
Lamb concentrates	1.62	1.98
Purchased forage	0.63	0.54
Fertilizer	4.15	3.85
Other forage costs	1.91	1.67
Total feed and forage	15.84	15.14
Vet and medicine	3.82	3.45
Miscellaneous and transport	2.99	2.84
Total variable costs	22.65	21.43
Gross margin	32.75	40.95
Gross margin per hectare	432	667

embarking on a new sheep enterprise is strongly recommended to seek the advice and knowledge of professional advisers. As we have seen, planning involves the assimilation of all the available information relative to the project and consulting professional specialists can often save a tremendous amount of time and money.

Planning aids

It has already been pointed out that factual information is required to fuel planning decisions involved with new enterprises or monitor

Table 1.3 Physical results for lowland spring lambing flocks, 1991. (Source: MLC, 1992a)

	Average	Top third
Lambs born alive per 100 ewes to ram	158	165
Lambs reared per 100 ewes to ram	152	159
Stocking rates		
Summer grazing	13.5	16.5
Overall grass	13.7	16.7
Overall grass and forage	13.2	16.3

Table 1.4 Contribution to the top third superiority in gross margin per hectare for two systems of production. (Source: MLC, 1992a)

	Lowland spring lambing	Upland
Stocking rate	54	77
Number of lambs reared	14	8
Lamb sale price per head	18	3
Flock replacement costs	5	12
Feed and forage costs	2	0
Other factors	7	0

existing ones. The data may relate to specific enterprises or be general information collated on an industry basis. In either case records must be kept in such a way as to be accessible and of potential value to sheep producers.

Enterprise data
In order to monitor the sheep enterprise, records of the important physical and financial parameters are required. These show whether the targets set at the beginning of the production year are being achieved and can thus highlight areas where remedial action is necessary. Enterprise data falls into two categories, dealing with the physical and financial aspects of the flock.

Physical performance

Records are needed of ewe numbers at key times in the year. Stock numbers need to be balanced so details of draft ewes sold out of the flock, replacements purchased or retained from the year's lamb crop, and any ewe deaths are required. Output measured by the number of lambs born, weaned and sold should be recorded. These figures permit the calculation of such factors as the number of lambs born per 100 ewes mated (referred to as 'lambing percentage') and the percentage of ewes barren – two fundamental measures of flock performance. Products of the flock should be recorded, including the weight of wool sold and the numbers of lambs sold at key times of the year. Weights and condition scores of ewes are also of value. In addition, movement of stock between different grazing areas should be recorded if the costs of grassland and forage crops are to be accurately allocated to the enterprise.

Financial performance

All financial transactions must be recorded so that a gross margin can be produced at the end of the sheep year. These are often the most difficult records to extract as they are inevitably bound up in the overall accounting system of the farm. When the time comes to gather together all these costs and items of income, backtracking over a period of twelve months can be a difficult and sometimes painful task. Large cost items such as fertilizer or concentrates may be itemized on invoices which included other major items for the farm, and some discipline and perseverance is required to extract the items pertaining specifically to the sheep enterprise. Other items such as the wool cheque or payments made for replacement ewes may be more easily accessible. Producers invariably remember these large items but neglect or lose track of the small costs which contribute to the final gross margin.

Recording the enterprise produces data on the physical and financial aspects of the flock which, when examined, can point the way to increased profitability or the more efficient use of resources. Generally this can be achieved through increasing output, by the better use of inputs or through the allocation of additional resources and an overall decrease in the unit costs of the enterprise. Increased output and decreased costs are often interlinked in such a way that the overall result is lower costs per unit of output.

Records provide the means of comparing flock performance levels against standards. Examination of the gross margin of the flock in this way will inevitably identify weak areas and any areas where an increased allocation of resources would be beneficial. Overall, records allow resources to be managed better.

Industry data
The accumulation of industry data requires the existence of a central agency to collate the information available from product sales such as lamb auction markets or slaughter houses. So, too, does the aggregation of enterprise data collected through an organised recording scheme. MLC serves this function in Britain through its economists and regional livestock consultants who provide individuals, industry bodies and national planning agencies with a wide range of valuable and informative data on the state of the sheep industry. The collection of market information on the number of slaughterings and the movement of sheep products is an invaluable aid for national planning. Factual up-to-the minute data enables short term forecasts to be made. Flockplan also fulfils a valuable industry role by taking individual enterprise data and collating it across systems of production. This data is then made widely available through periodic publications.

Industry data in Britain is available from sources other than MLC but these are more specific in nature. In Scotland, flock performance data is available from the Scottish Agricultural College who produce valuable technical bulletins which relate to specific sheep production topics. In England the Agricultural Development and Advisory Service (ADAS) fulfils a similar role. The University of Exeter, as part of an on-going exercise, collates sheep production data from University Agricultural Economics Departments throughout England and Wales every five years. Some valuable sheep data which complements Flockplan data is included in this sample.

Planning examples

Planned nutrition
The cyclical nature of sheep production, particularly in Britain, requires a detailed knowledge of the whole production cycle as decisions taken in one period of the year may have little bearing on the performance of the flock until many months later. Nutritional management through the year is one example of an essential planning element contributing to profitable production.

The standard of nutrition in the weeks before mating as well as during the mating period is important in determining the number of lambs conceived. Nutrition during pregnancy determines the number of lambs subsequently born alive at a birth weight which will ensure survival and the prospects of high growth. Ewe nutrition before and after lambing has a major effect on milk production and hence on lamb growth rate. Nutrition before and after weaning replenishes the body reserves utilized during pregnancy and early lactation and prepares the ewe for the next season's production.

It is, however, essential that ewe nutrition is considered on a year-round basis and no individual stage of production should be dealt with in isolation. If, for example, an attempt were made to increase the lamb crop by improving the standard of feeding before mating and no provision were made to cater for the increased number of lambs by improving nutrition during late pregnancy and lactation, the result could be disastrous. It is likely that lamb birth weights would be reduced, that a high proportion of lambs would die and that ewes would have insufficient milk to rear those lambs which did survive. In addition, there would probably be a reduction in the overall weight of lambs weaned and an increase in ewe mortality.

The continuous nature of production is emphasized by Fig. 1.2 which shows the changes in liveweight throughout the year relative to weight at mating for mature ewes. Ewe weight relative to mating

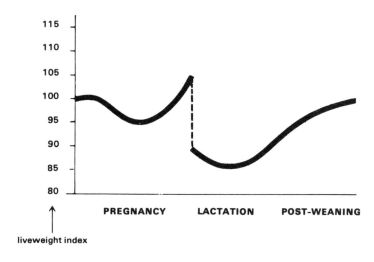

Fig. 1.2 Annual liveweight changes for mature ewes (100 = liveweight at mating). (Source: MLC, 1988a)

weight falls slightly in mid-pregnancy and then increases sharply due to foetal growth. This increase is greater for ewes bearing multiple litters. At parturition ewe weight drops considerably, continues to decline through lactation and it is not until weaning that the ewe has the opportunity to recover bodyweight. Feed resources have to be planned to match these ewe weight fluctuations through the year if serious and irreversible liveweight changes are to be avoided.

Planned grassland use
Grazing plays a large and important part in most sheep production systems. In Britain sheep not only graze grass but also utilize forage crops grown specifically to fill gaps in the availability of grass or graze stubbles and other by-products from arable crops. In situations where sheep are kept in conjunction with other grazing livestock and where arable crops are also grown, it is important to decide on the allocation of land to the various crops bearing in mind the grazing requirements of the animals likely to be kept. These decisions ought to be taken in the summer of the previous year, before the sowing of any winter cereals. If winter cereals are not grown the decisions can be delayed until later but they must be made before ploughing starts.

Several different sets of factors need to be taken into account when planning grassland requirements and usage. Firstly, the production potential of the land, rainfall, type of grassland available and level of nitrogen use envisaged can all be combined to estimate the amount of grass that can be grown. The numbers of stock, their size and the growth rate of young animals can be combined to give an idea of the grazing requirements of the animals to be kept. In addition, an estimate of the conservation requirements for the following winter should be taken into account. An example of the grazing requirements of a lowland flock is compared with the likely dry matter production from a typical grass sward in Fig. 1.3. When supply is in excess of demand, conservation or grazing with another species can take up the extra supply. In a period of deficit additional concentrates or conserved feed may be used, but this is to be avoided if at all possible because of the additional costs which will be incurred.

All these factors should, finally, be combined with an estimate of the land requirements of the other enterprises on the farm in order to maximise the financial returns from the farm as a whole. This is not a small task and the penalties for not planning correctly this far in advance can be substantial, even in terms of the sheep enterprise alone.

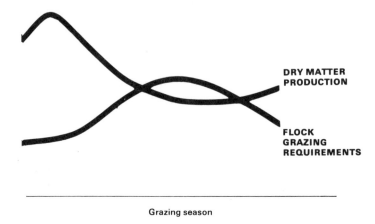

Grazing season

Fig. 1.3 Dry matter requirements of the lowland flock and grass production.

Consider the situation on an arable farm utilizing short term leys as a break crop. If it is the intention to finish all the lambs from the flock by the end of July, as is often the case in eastern England, considerable financial penalties may be incurred if there is not enough grass in June and July due to poor establishment the previous autumn or over-grazing in the spring. Insufficient grass will reduce the lamb growth rate through competition and lambs will thus be sold at a lower weight than necessary, perhaps losing as much as £2 per carcase, or concentrates will be required to maintain the anticipated growth at extra cost. Alternatively, lambs may be finished later in the season at a time when prices are lower. Whichever of the three solutions is adopted, the result will be a reduced level of profitability.

A planned lamb finishing enterprise
Not all lambs in Britain are sold for slaughter from the flock in which they were bred. There is an appreciable trade in lambs from breeding flocks to store lamb finishing enterprises. Store lamb finishing is often thought of as an enterprise for opportunists, relying on buying cheaply and selling when the market is right. Undoubtedly, this attitude may lead to success but margins are small and can easily be eroded by an unexpected feed bill or turn in the market. Losses in store lamb enterprises can be reduced, however, by taking into account the factors known to influence profitability and planning the system of feeding around them.

At the outset it is possible to estimate the maximum price that can be paid to buy in store lambs, given the cost of feeding, the weight gain and the anticipated price at sale. There are several options available for feeding store lambs according to the farm circumstances and the enterprise plan. In certain areas root crops are grown specifically for lamb finishing while in others reliance may be on grass finishing with some concentrate supplementation. The feeding regime chosen must be at a cost which will provide a reasonable feeders margin. A comparison of gross margins per lamb from average store lamb finishing systems to top third systems in 1987–8 highlights the importance of lamb purchase price and feed costs to the success of the system (Fig. 1.4). Success is achieved through buying lambs cheaply, selling well and keeping feed costs down.

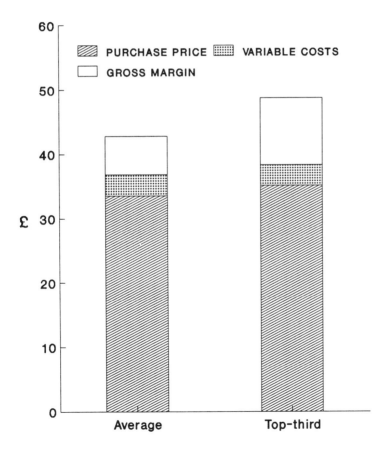

Fig. 1.4 Store lamb results in 1987–8 – components of lamb sale price. (Source: MLC, 1988c)

Planned flock health

Flock health is another aspect of sheep production where financial benefits can accrue if an effective plan is followed. For example, it is known that worm burdens which can build up in young lambs in May and June significantly depress performance, and the organisation of farm resources to provide clean grazing (i.e. grassland that has not been grazed by sheep in the previous year) for young lambs as a means of controlling these internal parasites can therefore be financially rewarding. A system incorporating clean grazing was developed by the then East of Scotland College of Agriculture (Rutter, 1983). It allows an increase in intensification without reducing lamb growth performance. The essential principle of the system is to identify the next year's clean grazing during the previous summer by finding fields being used for cereals, cattle, conservation or reseeding. Only cattle or dosed ewes should be kept on those areas until the end of the grazing season. During the following year sheep should be wormed immediately prior to being turned out on to the 'clean' grass. This should ensure a good level of protection for the sheep at grass.

An example of the system devised by Rutter with use with permanent pasture involving a three year cycle of sheep, hay and suckler cows is illustrated in Fig. 1.5. Finally, the choice of clean grazing system must depend upon the types of land and their proportions, field sizes and other physical considerations such as stock numbers.

This introductory chapter has presented a number of concepts and planning aids which will be referred to again in later sections dealing

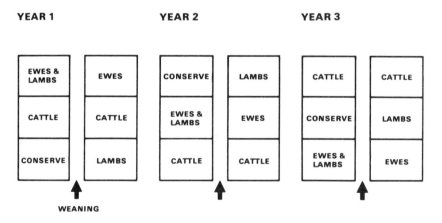

Fig. 1.5 A system of clean grazing for permanent pasture with conservation. (Source: Rutter, 1983)

with industry data and specific resources. It is most important that anyone contemplating a sheep enterprise understands the value of plans and budgets at the outset and calls on advisers with relevant experience wherever possible. Once an enterprise has been established, the value of some degree of monitoring as a means of assessing the degree to which targets initially set are met cannot be overstressed. Above all an understanding of the fundamental aspects of sheep production is essential if the available resources are to be fully exploited.

Section 1
Aspects of Production

Any view of sheep production will depend on the range of vision of the observer. Individual producers are generally only concerned with those aspects of production close to home such as the prices which relate to their products in the local or regional markets. Large scale operators and producers in countries where national aspects impinge more on their own enterprises will take a more distant view. Personnel involved in national or international planning must inevitably take a long range view of sheep production and absorb pertinent facts and statistics on a global basis.

In this section some consideration is given to the world's sheep population and the important products, with particular reference to aspects of world trade in wool and sheepmeat. Examples of the types of systems and environments are discussed to illustrate the diverse nature of the species and highlight some management and planning problems. Finally, the European sheep scene is examined in detail as a background to the British sheep industry under the CAP.

2 World Trade and Production

Sheep are found extensively throughout the world, from the arid desert areas to the cold regions of the northern and southern hemispheres. In its domesticated form the sheep is a multi-purpose species providing a diversity of products from a wide variety of breeds and sub-breeds. Sheep have evolved to meet the specific needs of the people for whom they provide for within a wide range of environments. In global terms sheep farming is predominantly aimed at wool production, particularly in the southern hemisphere. However, meat production is the major product in Britain and therefore forms the basis for much of this book.

It is in recognition of the diverse nature of the species that the following chapter is devoted to a general overview of world sheep production. Readers unfamiliar with the sheep industry in Britain will, it is hoped, find a reference point from which to explore the fundamental planning issues discussed and will relate them to their own particular situation.

The world sheep population

Latest estimates by the Food and Agriculture Organisation of the United Nations (FAO) put the world sheep population at 1190 million (FAO, 1991), which makes sheep the third most numerous species of farm animal after chickens and cattle. The summary of world animal statistics shown in Table 2.1 indicates that Asia has the largest sheep population, representing 28% of the world population. Oceania, i.e. Australia, New Zealand and the Pacific Islands, has the next largest population (19% of the world total), followed by Africa (16%), the former USSR (12%), Europe (13%), South America (9%) and North and Central America (2%). However, these figures do not reveal the full importance of sheep production in the various continents and

Table 2.1 World population of farm animals by region in 1990. (000,000 head) (Source: FAO, 1991)

	Africa	North and Central America	South America	Asia	Europe	Oceania	USSR	World
Sheep	205.1	19.2	112.6	338.2	152.2	226.1	137.0	1190.5
Cattle	187.8	160.1	263.9	393.9	124.0	31.3	118.4	1279.3
Pigs	13.6	88.8	55.6	432.6	181.9	5.3	78.9	856.8
Goats	173.9	13.9	23.4	322.0	15.4	2.0	6.5	557.0
Chickens	861.0	1945.0	933.0	4447.0	1271.0	84.0	1200.0	10740.0
Turkeys	6.0	102.0	10.0	11.0	79.0	2.0	47.0	257.0
Ducks	17.0	15.0	11.0	493.0	38.0	—	—	573.0
Horses	5.0	14.1	14.3	16.9	4.2	0.5	5.9	60.9
Mules	1.4	3.7	3.3	6.1	0.4	—	<0.1	14.8
Asses	13.0	3.7	4.0	21.5	1.0	<0.1	0.3	43.6
Buffaloes	2.5	<0.1	1.2	136.2	0.4	—	0.4	140.8
Camels	14.5	—	—	4.6	—	—	0.3	19.4

countries of the world. When the density of sheep per unit area is considered Europe, with 13% of the world's sheep population, is shown as the most densely populated area of the world with 31 sheep per 100 ha of land and 183 sheep per 100 ha of permanent pasture (Table 2.2). On this basis of comparison, Asia is only the third most densely populated with 12 sheep per 100 ha of land and 50 sheep per 100 ha of permanent pasture.

An alternative method of comparison based on the number of sheep to man is presented in the final column of Table 2.2. This shows the extremely high ratio found in Oceania of just over eight hundred and sixty sheep per head of population, with the former USSR, South America and Africa having the next highest density indices. The role of the various countries in world trade is discussed later in this chapter and it is interesting to note that two of these areas, Oceania and South America, are heavily involved in the export of sheep products.

While these figures are of considerable interest when trying to put sheep production into a world context, some care must be taken in their interpretation. Many countries provide only estimates of their sheep population, and of those that collect accurate census data many do so at different times of the year and hence at different points in the annual production cycle.

The statistics presented in Table 2.1 only relate to one year, and trends in world numbers over recent years for the more important sheep populations are also worth considering. In Table 2.3 figures are given for the world as a whole and also for the eleven countries with

Table 2.2 World sheep density indices, 1990. (Source: FAO, 1991)

	Sheep per 100 ha of land	Sheep per 100 ha of permanent pasture	Sheep per 100 head of population
Africa	7	23	33
North and Central America	1	5	5
South America	6	23	39
Asia	12	50	11
Europe	31	183	31
Oceania	27	52	861
USSR	6	37	48
World	9	36	23

Table 2.3 Changes in sheep populations of the world in major sheep keeping countries, 1981–90. (Source: FAO, 1991)

	Numbers in 000,000 head			% of world population in 1990
	1981	1990	% change	
World	1130.8	1190.5	+5	100
USSR	141.6	137.0	−3	12
Australia	133.4	167.8	+26	14
China	105.2	113.5	+8	10
New Zealand	71.2	58.3	−18	5
India	41.5	54.6	+32	5
Turkey	48.6	31.5	−35	3
Iran	34.4	34.0	−1	3
South Africa	31.7	32.6	+3	3
UK	32.3	29.5	−9	2
Argentina	30.0	28.6	−5	2
Pakistan	28.5	29.2	+2	2
				61

the largest sheep populations which together accounted for 61% of the world's sheep population in 1990. The 5% increase in the world's sheep population between 1981 and 1990 conceals several interesting trends in individual countries. The most extreme changes over this nine year period were in India where the population increased by 32% and in Turkey where there was a decrease of 35%. The considerable growth in Asia is a result of the 'green revolution' while sheep numbers have declined in other countries as a direct result of competition from more profitable enterprises. Australian numbers which fell in the period between 1971 and 1981 due to unfavourable wool prices in the mid 1970s and to severe drought conditions in more recent years, had recovered by 1990. Such changes in an individual country's sheep population reflect the dynamic nature of the industry and show how industries can react to both international and national influences. These movements appear to occur irrespective of whether the economy in question is managed centrally, as was the case in many eastern European countries, or whether the industry depends on the combined efforts of a mass of individual producers.

The contribution of any single sheep industry to the world trade in sheep products does not necessarily depend upon either the size of its sheep population or the amounts of any one product produced. For example, production from the relatively large sheep populations of Africa, Asia and the former USSR referred to earlier has little effect on world trade because their products are in great demand on their local home markets. These countries, therefore, have little impact on the supply and demand situation of world production.

In the long term, however, world trade may be increasingly influenced by these areas. Eastern European countries are intent on achieving self-sufficiency in sheep products. These intentions, coupled with a growing demand from the Middle East and south east Asia for sheepmeat, may well affect world trade in the long term.

Sheep products

Four primary products of sheep can be identified: wool, sheepmeat, milk and skins (Table 2.4). Wool dominates the world trade in sheep products because its production is concentrated in the southern hemisphere where the demand for wool is limited. In most of the wool producing areas sheepmeat is a secondary product, i.e. mutton from Australia and South Africa and lamb from New Zealand. Sheepmeat production is dominant in northern Europe and the Middle East, with wool or hair as the secondary product. Milk production on a large scale is mainly found in Mediterranean areas where meat or wool or both are of secondary importance. Milk is also an important product in other areas, particularly Asia, but here it is mostly consumed at home. Skin production is found in a number of widely different situations.

Wool production
The total percentage of wool used for textiles has shown a dramatic decline in the past thirty years, but this has been almost entirely due to the increasing supply of synthetic fibres and the total weight of wool produced has in fact remained fairly static. The contribution of wool now appears to have stabilized at approximately 5% of total fibre production (Table 2.5). Recently, however, the demand for 'natural' products has raised the demand for woollen garments particularly in developed countries.

With the exception of the former USSR, the major wool producers are all in the southern hemisphere while five of the six major importers

Table 2.4 Production of sheep products by region in 1990 (000 t). (Source: FAO, 1991)

	Africa	North and Central America	South America	Asia	Europe	Oceania	USSR	World
Wool (scoured)	131	27	202	276	197	983	283	2096
Mutton and lamb	864	204	286	1987	1416	1163	950	6871
Sheep's milk	1376	—	35	3385	3598	—	75	8470
Sheepskins	174	23	84	426	231	275	131	1344

Table 2.5 World fibre production – % share of textile market. (Source: International Wool Secretariat, 1992)

	Clean wool	Synthetic	Cellulosics	Cotton	Flax
1951	9	1	15	70	5
1961	9	5	17	65	4
1971	6	23	14	54	3
1981	5	35	10	48	2
1990 (p)	5	38	7	48	2

(p) provisional

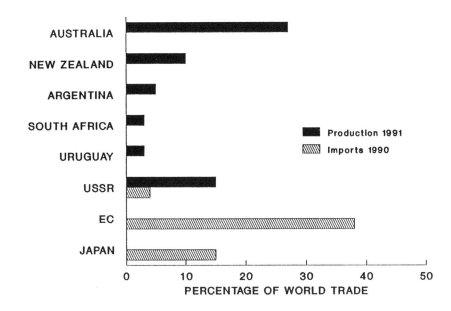

Fig. 2.1 World wool production and imports. (Source: International Wool Secretariat, 1992)

of wool are in Europe. The former USSR is unique in that it is both a major producer and a major importer of wool. Percentages of world production and imports are summarized in Fig. 2.1.

Wool can be classified according to whether it is produced as a main product or as a by-product to meat (Ponting, 1980). Where wool is the main product a further subdivision into fine wools and coarse carpet wools can be made. Merino sheep, which predominate in the southern hemisphere, are the major source of the fine wools used entirely for garments whereas carpet wools are found mainly in Asia. Wool produced from sheep bred primarily for meat is often referred to as 'crossbred wool' and accounts for over half the total world wool production. New Zealand, with its large quantities of Romney wool, is regarded as the major producer of crossbred wool. Production trends for the three main wool types in recent years are presented in Table 2.6.

Sheepmeat production
The international trade in sheepmeat is active in both the carcase and the live animal sectors, with Australia and New Zealand dominating

Table 2.6 World clean wool production (000 000 kg). (Source: International Wool Secretariat, 1983)

	1960	1970	1980	1982
Merino	560	604	622	641
Crossbred	627	706	560	544
Other (mainly carpet)	293	295	428	440
Total	1480	1605	1610	1625

supply and Europe and Japan creating the strongest demand. Sheepmeat produced in Asia, Africa and the former USSR is mainly for home consumption although in the Middle East a strong trade exists between neighbouring countries, particularly for live sheep.

Sheepmeat products can be divided into mutton and lamb, with the production and consumption of lamb being most important in Europe. Britain dominates the European demand for lamb and receives a significant proportion of her annual consumption in frozen carcase meat from New Zealand, the largest supplier of lamb in the world market (Fig. 2.2). Australia, on the other hand, dominates world supplies of mutton although the volume of carcases has been reduced in recent years in favour of live exports, particularly to the Middle East. Wool, as we have seen, is the major product from Australian flocks but the environment and the large Merino stocks so suited to wool production combine to create a considerable surplus of mature sheep.

The world trade in sheepmeat is summarized in Table 2.7. The Middle East, where there is a strong demand because of the religious ban on pork meat and pork products, is an expanding market. In addition to the considerable imports of carcase meat in the Middle East, over four million head of live sheep were exported to the area from Australia in 1991.

There is great variation in lamb carcase weights produced on world markets due to the many breeds and crosses involved in lamb production. In Britain, for example, small Welsh Mountain ewes maintained in the upland and mountain areas of Wales produce purebred lambs with a potential carcase weight of 8–12 kg whereas the much larger North Country Cheviot ewes kept in upland areas of the North of Scotland are capable of producing carcases of 19–22 kg. Management practices may also influence carcase weight. Small carcases

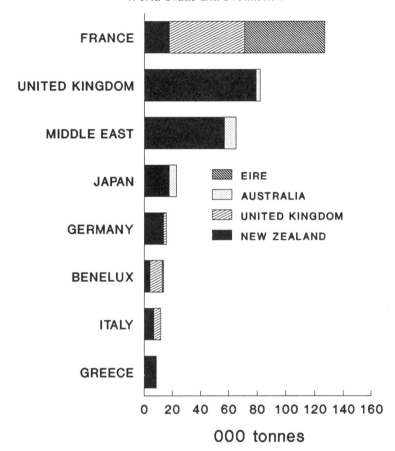

Fig. 2.2 Major markets for lamb carcase meat in 1991. (Source: MLC, 1992c)

similar to those produced by the Welsh Mountain ewe are derived from the early slaughter of young lambs from milking ewe flocks in Mediterranean areas. In general, carcase weights produced in European countries vary considerably as a result of the different breeds and management systems employed. It is virtually impossible to define one weight as preferable to another.

Unlike the majority of other meats, sheepmeat undergoes little processing between the producer and consumer, the carcase not being broken down into final joints until it reaches the butcher's shop. In recent years European demand for lamb has declined and this fall in lamb consumption has caused some concern, particularly in Britain. Recent consumer surveys have revealed that the British housewife

Table 2.7 World trade in sheepmeat 1991 (000 t). (Source: MLC, 1992c)

| | Exporting Countries | | | |
| | Australia | | New Zealand | |
	Lamb	Mutton	Lamb	Mutton
Total exports	38.3	191.6	292.8	84.1
Of which to				
Middle East	8.1	60.9	63.9	
EC	4.3		149.7	25.6
(United Kingdom)			(79.2)	(16.2)
(Greece)			(9.0)	(4.0)
Japan	5.2	26.2	17.9	5.0
S Korea				14.3
N America			15.2	

considers lamb to be fatty, wasteful and lacking in versatility. The problem of fatness has been tackled by producers and there has been a considerable reduction in carcase fatness since the introduction of the EC sheepmeat regime. However, fatness is only one of the problems associated with lamb and careful consideration of butchery techniques has been necessary in order to overcome other associated problems of consumer resistance.

Conventional lamb cutting entails the division of the carcase into a number of primal joints from which either leg and shoulder joints or loin and best end chops are taken (Fig. 2.3). These joints all contain bone, considered by many to be the major cause of waste and creating carving difficulties, particularly in the shoulder joint. New butchery techniques have been developed by MLC meat technicians to overcome the problems of these conventional cuts. These involve the complete de-boning of sides of lamb from which either rolled joints or steaks and chops can then be prepared. These new cuts, which complement the traditional forms of presentation, are attractive, convenient in size and easy to cook and carve. Saleable yields from boneless sides of lamb at the same weight and fat level and prepared by two different methods are presented in Table 2.8.

The retail prices of the new cuts have to reflect the fact that the meat contains no bone and that appreciable excess fat has been trimmed away. The higher cost focuses the consumer's attention on the

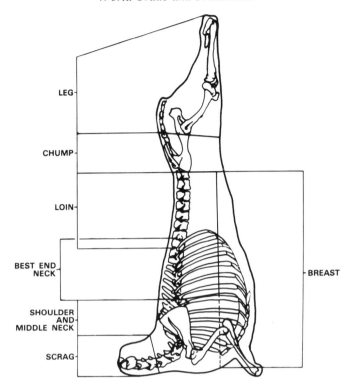

Fig. 2.3 Conventional cuts of lamb in Britain. (Source: MLC, 1980a)

attractiveness of the cut and as the development of the technique has progressed it has become quite clear than lean lambs are required. The new methods of cutting and presentation are unable to hide high fat levels which make the cuts look less attractive.

The new technique can be carried out on a wide weight range of lambs. Light and medium weight lambs (10–19 kg) are suited to the boneless roll method while heavier carcases (above 19 kg) are particularly suited to the steaking method. The new cuts have been well received by all sectors of the industry and these methods have become widely adopted, particularly in the large multiple outlets.

Although in general sheepmeat undergoes little processing between producer and consumer, curing does occur in certain locations. Smoked Icelandic lamb is one example, providing an excellent alternative to fresh lamb, while in east Norway salted leg of lamb *fenalår* is a traditional method of curing. In the United Kingdom the Highlands and Islands Development Board have been considering various ways

Table 2.8 Saleable yields from boneless sides of lamb prepared by two different methods (% side weight). (Source: MLC, 1983)

	Boneless rolled joints	Steaks and joints
Steaks	—	21.9
Boneless chops	—	10.4
Rolled joints	66	27.4
Lean trim	5	9.1
Kidney	0.5	0.5
Total saleable meat	71.5	69.3
Fat trim	7.8	9.3
Bone and waste	20	19.4
Cutting loss	0.7	2

of curing lamb as a means of developing trade in the remoter areas of Scotland.

Milk production

The large quantities of milk produced in Africa and Asia are mainly for home consumption and it is only in the Mediterranean area that milk is regarded as a major product of the ewe. The largest share of milk output is used for manufacturing cheese: soft cream cheese of the *feta* type in the eastern Mediterranean which compensates for a low output from dairy cattle, and aged-cheese in the western Mediterranean. Roquefort is the best known of the latter variety and is produced in the south-west of France from Lacaune ewes. Cheese production of this kind is well suited to small family farms and has tended increasingly to cater for a luxury market. This type of production is, however, susceptible to market forces and depends to a large extent on the successful development of the market. Recently unit size has been increasing and development has been along lines similar to dairy cow production.

In this connection, the recent formation of an association of sheep milk producers in Britain points to a growing market for ewe milk products. Readers in the UK interested in this aspect are referred to a specialist book dealing with the subject in some depth (Mills, 1989).

Sheepskins

Although often neglected, sheepskins and in particular those from lambs provide a valuable product and feature significantly in world trade. Processing without removal of the wool gives a dressed skin suitable for manufacture into clothing and rugs, while wool removal and subsequent tanning provides a valuable leather. This latter process is centred in Mazament in south-western France. World trade in sheepskins is dominated by the larger sheep economies of Australia and New Zealand, with a contribution from Asia. The majority of the skins are salted, semi-processed and exported to Europe. In Britain, skin production is a small part of the output from the ewe flock but the market value of the skin is supportive within the overall industry context and should not be ignored. Care and attention on the farm when vaccinating stock and careful handling will minimize skin damage and is to be commended as responsible practice.

A few breeds have been developed to produce special skins or pelts, and in these flocks skin is the major product. The most important of these specialized pelt sheep is the Karakul of which there are reported to be some 12.5 million in the former Soviet Socialist Republics of Uzbekistan and Turkmenistan, the main centres of production. Lambs are killed soon after birth to produce Astrakhan or Persian lamb skins. A number of other breeds produce valuable grey or black pelts, including the Romanov in the former USSR, the Gotland in Sweden, the Wrzosowka in Poland and coloured variants of the Icelandic breed. Skin production accounts for over half of total producer returns in Swedish Gotland flocks from which the valuable fleeces are specially tanned and made into attractive garments.

Secondary products

The integration of a ewe flock into an intensive farm structure provides a high level of soil fertility and this is considered by many to outweigh the major products of meat or wool. Continuous cereal producers on the light downland soils of the southern parts of England have received considerable benefits from the introduction of a grassland break and grazing ewes. Although recent agronomic developments have also contributed, there is little doubt that sheep are a significant factor. In addition to increased cereal yields, the structure of the soil has also improved and has a more friable structure for tillage which assists seed bed preparation and certain cultivations.

Systems and environments

Europe

Within Europe the most important species of farm animal are cattle, followed by pigs and then sheep. The sheep population in Europe, half of which is located in the twelve member countries of the EC, accounts for 13% of the total world population. Two countries dominate the European sheep population in terms of trade – the United Kingdom which dominates the export trade and France which is the main market for imports of sheepmeat. The EC sheepmeat regime regulates sheepmeat trade within the EC and, to a certain extent the trade with other countries. Sheep production within the EC and in particular within the UK will be discussed in Chapter 3.

Spain

Although famous as the home of the Merino, the world's most important wool producing breed, Spain has had little impact on European sheep production. Ewe flocks are run extensively across stubbles and arable by-products, herded by day and returned to folds at night. The majority of Spanish breeds, such as Manchega and Araganese, have extensive breeding seasons with the result that lambing often lasts from autumn through to spring. Little effort seems to be put into concentrating lambing into one period. Transhumance, the practice of moving sheep from dry lowland areas to the green hillier mountain pastures during summer, still survives.

Products from the Spanish sheep industry are varied. In certain areas to the south of Madrid dairy flocks, predominantly of the Manchega breed, are found and significant volumes of small lambs are produced. Spanish taste in sheepmeat is for small, fat-free carcases of around 12 kg which are most often the product of dairy flocks. Little emphasis is placed on wool production despite the predominance of the Merino. Technical improvements are possible and a number have been attempted, but the organization of the industry is fragmented and innovation appears to be a matter left to individuals.

On one large estate, for example, considerable investment was made in irrigation equipment to increase output per hectare. In conjunction with this scheme, large terminal sire breeds were imported from the UK, France and Germany to increase carcase weights produced from the indigenous ewe breeds. At the same time high yielding Awassi dairy ewes were imported from Israel to increase milk output from the dairy flock. These moves were technically successful but the irrigated pastures enriched by highly stocked sheep became so productive that because of external economic pressures arable and cash crops were grown instead. The ewe flocks are now managed on higher, poorer ground where irrigation is not yet possible. Good planning and execution can, therefore, be too successful.

The large carcases being produced were not well received by Spanish consumers and in reality the potential of the larger terminal sire breeds was never fully exploited. The initiative of individuals continues, however, with one producer investing considerable amounts of time and money to increase flock output by increasing the number of lambs sold per ewe per year. This is being done through a large selection programme involving 3000 breeding ewes. Two criteria, litter size and lambing interval, are being measured, with top rams selected on the basis of a selection index.

Since the entry of Spain into the EC the level of exports from the UK to the Spanish market has increased steadily. In particular, light hill lambs from Scotland and Wales are acceptable to the consumers as alternatives to the light Spanish lambs. MLC is actively promoting the development of this market.

Norway
In contrast to Spain, animal production is an important sector of the agricultural economy in Norway, with milk production dominating the livestock sector. However, the majority of the land area (approximately 70%) is above the tree line. Of Norway's total land area, only 3% is arable and 27% is in productive forest. Lowland areas of the general European type do not exist. The large tracts of mountainous pasture found in many districts are of considerable value to sheep producers and consequently sheep production is in a favourable position. Norwegian farmers, particularly those in northern and western areas, divide their efforts between fishing, farming and forestry to create a worthwhile income. Because of this and the sparse population in many areas, agricultural policy is an integral part of the government's economic, regional and food policies.

Average flock size is small – about thirty-five breeding ewes – and the majority of flocks are housed throughout the winter. The management of the breeding flocks reflects the difficult topography of the country and the harshness and severity of the climate, particularly during the winter months. Traditionally, agricultural communities would spend the winter months at homesteads in the valleys and in May move their families and stock to the mountain pastures where they would stay for the whole summer. Mountain villages or *seters* above the tree line were a common feature of the mountain scenery. In recent years, however, this practice has disappeared, and families now tend to stay in the valleys with only the stock being sent to the mountains.

The vast mountainous grazing areas are covered with snow until the end of May and the size of the flocks is therefore limited to the carrying capacity of the in-bye ground in the valleys. Ewes and lambs are turned out to the mountains in the spring and left unattended throughout the summer period until early autumn when they are brought down for mating and subsequent inwintering. An advantage to the ewe and lamb is that as the snow line recedes, exposed vegetation commences growth. In effect, strip grazing occurs with the animals benefiting from the fresh regrowth. The majority of the lambs are slaughtered over the autumn period at an average carcase weight of 18 kg.

Argentina

The semi-arid grasslands typical of much of Patagonia make arable cropping unprofitable in that region. However, large estates grazing cattle and sheep are common. The Estancia Condor is one such estate, occupying 200 000 ha in the south-eastern corner of Santa Cruz province and reaching almost down to the Straits of Magellan, a latitude of 52°S. The estate runs 100 000 sheep and 2000 head of cattle. The sheep are a locally produced breed called the Cormo Argentino, derived from an extensive crossing programme involving the Australia Cormo, Peppin Merino and Corriedale breeds. The Cormo Argentino produces a fine quality wool with a long staple, suitable for producing high quality garments. It produces a heavier fleece than either of the two main parent breeds and a carcase suited to lamb or mutton production. The Cormo Argentino is well adapted to the environment of southern Argentina and because of the extensive nature of the system under which it is kept has several 'easy-care' properties. These include having no horns, skin wrinkles or wool on the face.

The Estancia Condor sells three main products: wool, meat and breeding stock. The decision to develop the Cormo Argentino was taken as a direct response to changing market conditions. The export trade in wool from Argentina to the more developed countries of the world demanded a higher quality wool with the emphasis on fineness, softness and an extremely white colour. This is the market at which the Cormo Argentino is aimed. Surplus lambs from the flock are sold at

10–12 kg carcase weight for export to Italy, and there is also a thriving trade in surplus breeding rams.

The extensive nature of the production system is a response to the soil conditions, rainfall and grazing potential of the indigenous grass species. On parts of the estate the annual rainfall is about 300 mm and here the ewes can be stocked at one per hectare. Fifty miles away the rainfall is much less and the stocking rate has to be reduced to 0.5 ewe/ha. On some parts of the estate a reseeding programme has been carried out using imported grass species and on those areas stocking rate has been increased to three times its traditional level. Reseeding requires a considerable amount of extra labour and capital, and under these conditions the initial problem in such a programme is the generation of enough spare cash to start the reseeding cycle.

United States of America
Sheep production in the United States has shown a marked decline in the last thirty-five years. Since 1958 there has been a fall in the sheep population from around thirty-one million to just below eleven million in 1990. High losses from predators have been a major cause. It has been estimated that in 1982 over one million animals were lost in this way. Marketing and distribution difficulties coupled with some consumer resistance are also contributary factors in this decline. The reduction in numbers has resulted in slaughter plant closures and this, together with lower supply, has fuelled the downwards spiral and inevitably weakened the competitive position of lamb with other red meats.

The ewe population is concentrated in the western states on either side of the Rocky Mountain chain running from Canada down to Mexico. In these areas flocks are quite large and run extensively over rough conditions. Ewe productivity is low (lambing percentages are in the range 75–125) and together with the loss to predators, the main loss is from lamb mortality. Low winter and spring temperatures coupled with high wind speeds are lethal to the new born lamb, and many flocks are now managed with a view to indoor lambing. This has proved profitable in terms of lamb sales per ewe, and increases of up to 98% have been reported. Flocks are dual purpose, with wool and meat providing the main income to the flock. The most common ewe breeds in these areas are the Columbia and Rambouillet, and significant proportions are mated to larger terminal sire breeds such as the Suffolk or Hampshire. Lambs are moved into feedlots and finished on forages and cereals.

Sheep production in the remaining areas of the USA is in small flocks where meat is the primary product.

USSR

The former USSR was one of the largest sheep producers in the world and a wide variety of systems and breeds were used within the country. Information about the Kaztalowsky State Farm was presented at the 1982 European Grassland Federation meeting in Reading (Corrall, 1983). The farm is situated in the Ural region of Kazakhstan which is characterized by about 200 mm of rainfall, 120 frost-free days and 110 days of snow per year. Temperatures range from −37°C to 40°C with January and July averages of −12°C and 23.9°C respectively. The light chestnut soils maintain local pasture species of the wormwood grass and saltwort type. The farm of 137 000 ha contains 127 000 ha of grassland of which 17% is used for hay making. This grassland carries 29 286 sheep, 1479 cattle, 387 horses and 16 camels.

The sheep are of the fine wool Merino type and are kept for meat as well as wool. The ewes average 4.1 kg of wool and produce 0.98 lambs/ewe which are killed at 40 kg liveweight. The sheep are managed on a nomadic system within the farm area during the grazing season and return to the main farmsteads for the winter. Under these conditions ewes are stocked at approximately 0.2 per hectare during the summer. The system is characterized by low inputs but the level of output is enough to provide a reasonable return on money invested.

With the break up of the former USSR and the move towards a free market the whole structure of the sheep industry in the new states will be under review.

Sudan

Sudan contains the third largest sheep population in Africa, after South Africa and Ethiopia. Production systems range from the very intensive grazing of irrigated forages along the River Nile to nomadic grazing in the west which relies on natural rain fed pastures. In the Blue Nile province annual rainfall ranges from 400 to 600 mm per year, occuring between June and October. During this rainy season the natural grasses show prolific growth and as the soil dries out they persist as standing hay until grazed. Temperatures range from 10°C in January to 40°C in April with daily averages of 20°C and 35°C respectively. Under these conditions sheep must have the ability to forage widely, withstand high temperatures, utilize water efficiently and exist on their body reserves for some months. Sudan desert sheep which exhibit these characteristics are hair sheep rather than wool sheep.

Village flocks in the Blue Nile area are taken out to graze the natural vegetation during the day and returned to their pens at night. The very young lambs remain in the village during the day and hence are only able to suckle at night. Although the ewes have the ability to lamb all through the year, successful matings tend to occur when the prevailing nutritional status of the ewe allows. Consequently the largest lamb crop occurs in January and February due to the effects of good grass growth during the rainy season. Unfortunately, lambs born at this time then have to endure five months of hot weather and poor nutrition until the next rainy season. Under these conditions lambs reach marketable weight (40 kg liveweight) at about two years of age (Pollott, 1979). Since this is the main source of income from such flocks, the physical environment clearly exerts considerable pressure on the profitability of the enterprise.

In the same area of Sudan large-scale irrigation schemes have been developed for the production of arable crops such as cotton, peanuts, sisal, sesame and sugar cane. More intensive systems of sheep production have been developed utilizing both the byproducts of these arable crops and irrigated forage crops as a break crop in the arable rotation. In these systems the same type of desert sheep as are kept in the village system perform well to produce a 40 kg lamb at nine months of age when fed in a feedlot, ten months of age under irrigated grazing and fourteen months of age when lambs reared on rain-fed grazing are finished under feedlot conditions.

The systems and environments covered in this chapter emphasize the diverse nature of sheep production around the world. In the majority of situations animal resources are exploited to the limits the environment allows. Manipulation of feed resources can overcome these restrictions but requires the provision of further resources such as capital investment, more labour and additional land. For example, increased output could be achieved in the extensive systems in Sudan if capital investment were available for irrigation equipment to provide increased forage supplies at critical times. Alternatively investment in feed lot facilities and additional expensive cereal feeds could improve productivity.

While increased output is technically possible in most situations, the decision to implement these innovations and convert a low input/low output system into a high input/high output system cannot be taken lightly. Careful planning and assessment of all the contributing factors is required.

3 United Kingdom Production Statistics

Market supply and the demand for sheep products will dictate world prices, thereby impinging on the domestic economy of a nation and influencing decisions made by individual producers. There is little the individual can do to influence these trends. While an understanding of the global trade in sheepmeat or wool is valuable, the prices in local markets and facts concerning trade in the area are more likely to influence a producer's policy decisions. Indeed quick access to market statistics in the local area may well influence even his day to day decision making. For example, a sheep producer in central England with the opportunity to market slaughter lambs at several centres can watch daily price trends at each centre and arrange his marketing to maximize the return per lamb. Sheep production statistics on a national level are clearly, then, essential for sensible decision making and an important element in the planning process.

This chapter is devoted to UK sheep production statistics in order to illustrate the information considered relevant and also to set the scene for material in later chapters which draws on the UK industry. Some reference is made, in passing, to the EC sheep population and industry since sheep in the UK are an integral and important part of this wider community. As was noted in chapter 2, the sheep population of Europe represents 13% of the total world sheep population and more than 70% of that is accounted for by the twelve member states of the EC.

EC sheep production

The sheep population of the EC in 1990 numbered over one hundred and eight million out of which, it has been estimated, there were some 72.1 million breeding ewes. Five countries accounted for the majority of these: UK (20%), France (12%), Greece (10%), Italy (11%) and

Spain (24%). With the exception of Eire, with 6%, none of the remainder had more than 3% of the ewe population (Table 3.1).

In view of its significant proportion of ewes, it is hardly surprising that the UK produces 33% of the community's sheepmeat, 36% of its wool and 26% of its sheepskin. Spain is the second largest producer with 19%, 16% and 27% respectively and in addition produces 10% of the EC's sheep's milk. France is a significant producer of meat, wool and skins but in particular produces 40% of the EC's sheep's milk, most of which is used in the manufacture of cheese.

It is interesting that of the four major sheep products only sheepmeat has been subject to regulation under the Common Agricultural Policy of the EC. Wool is considered to be an industrial product and therefore exempt. Sheepskins are never seen as part of the producer's return, more often being the product of the slaughterhouse, and sheep's milk is confined to the Mediterranean countries where long established markets for the product exist.

The EC sheepmeat regime

As part of the Common Agricultural Policy of member states, the EC sheepmeat regime came into effect on 20 October 1980 in an attempt to achieve a single community price for sheepmeat. The French sheep industry was only about 79% self-sufficient in sheepmeat, and because the amount of chilled lamb which can be imported is limited under the voluntary restraint agreements to 'sensitive areas' there is a high demand for fresh lamb. High prices in the French market attracted sheepmeat from the UK and Ireland, but from the time that these two countries joined the EC in 1973 until the introduction of the CAP the French market had been protected by a system of import licences and import duties. The system was eventually challenged in 1977 as being contrary to the Treaty of Rome and was replaced with a bilateral agreement between France and Ireland. This was eventually ruled as being illegal in 1979, just prior to the introduction of the sheepmeat regime.

The sheepmeat regime can be divided into four important areas: internal market support, annual ewe premiums, trade with non-EC countries and miscellaneous factors such as currency, less favoured areas, etc.

Internal market support

Internal market support measures were introduced covering the regulation of prices, the provision of private storage aid, intervention

Table 3.1 Sheep population and production in the EC, 1990. (Source: Adapted from FAO, 1991 and MLC, 1992c)

	Numbers (millions)		Products (000 t)			
	Total sheep	Breeding ewes	Sheepmeat	Wool	Milk	Skins
EC Total	108.1	72.1	1185	205.8	2.7	168.1
% from						
Belgium and Luxembourg	<1	<1	<1	<1		1
Denmark	<1	<1	<1	<1		<1
Germany	4	3	5	12		4
Greece	10	10	11	4	24	9
France	11	12	15	11	40	10
Irish Republic	5	6	7	8		9
Italy	11	11	5	7	23	10
Netherlands	2	2	3	1		1
UK	27	20	33	36		26
Portugal	5	3	2	4	3	3
Spain	25	24	19	16	10	27

buying and variable premium support. Member states were given the choice to opt for intervention buying or a variable premium scheme as a means for market support but only France and the UK took up this option. France chose an intervention system, while the UK opted for a variable premium scheme which remained in use for over a decade from the introduction of the scheme in October 1980 until January 1992.

The variable premium scheme was only operated in Great Britain throughout this period, Northern Ireland having opted out in 1983. An annual scale of guide prices was set at the beginning of the marketing year (1 April). When the average market price was below the weekly guide price, a premium equal to the difference was paid on all eligible sheep marketed, either liveweight or deadweight, in that week. Lambs were certified as eligible for this variable premium on the basis of their weight, fat cover and conformation.

Lambs and carcases from Great Britain for export to member states carried a charge equal to the appropriate variable premium for the week, as the 'clawback'. Exports to non-EC countries were exempt from clawback. The guaranteed return provided for by the variable premium scheme and its associated pattern of guide prices proved invaluable for producers in their planning decisions.

The sheepmeat regime was revised in 1991 and the variable premium and associated clawback payments were phased out before complete removal from 6 January 1992. The intervention system which had only applied in France was widened and became a private storage scheme operating in any member state including Great Britain. The scheme provides a safety net to support the market should prices fall below a minimum level but to date the uptake has been small.

The annual premium
An EC basic price for fresh and chilled sheep carcases is set annually by the EC Council of Agricultural Ministers. The levels set take into account the various factors including the current and forecast sheep marketing situation, production costs and the market situation in other sectors, particularly beef and veal. The basic price is subject to seasonal adjustments on a weekly basis. The actual basic price applied also depends on the application of a European Community Budgetary Stabilizer for sheepmeat which was a mechanism introduced in 1988 to limit expenditure on the overall sheepmeat regime.

The basis of the mechanism is a 'threshold flock' the size of which is set by the European Commission. A threshold flock of 18.1 million ewes has been set for Great Britain and 45.3 million ewes for the rest of the EC in total. The mechanism works in such a way that for every 1% by which this threshold is exceeded, there is a 1% reduction in the basic price which then leads to a cut in the annual ewe premium. In recent years the cuts in the basic price at the end of each marketing year have always been offset by green rate devaluations which in effect has meant little net change.

It is on the basis of the basic price that market returns are monitored and annual ewe premiums made to compensate for any income loss to producers. Annual premiums which were regionally based prior to 1992 are now differentiated on two production systems; light lamb production where the primary output is milk or milk products plus associated lamb carcases of 5–6 kg, and specialist heavy lamb production. The annual ewe premium paid to light lamb producers is 70% of the calculated annual ewe premium for heavy lamb producers.

A community average price is calculated for monitoring purposes in relation to the sheepmeat private storage aid scheme and for the determination of the income loss element in the calculation of the annual ewe premium. Following a review of the sheepmeat regime in 1991 price reporting in all member states is based on a standard quality for fresh or chilled carcases. The standard price derived for each member state is then weighted by a coefficient which relates to its share of total EC production to give the community average price. In Great Britain a standard quality quotation is derived from lambs in the standard and medium weights categories (32.1–45.5 kg liveweight).

From 1990 payment of the annual ewe premium has been limited with full payment only being made on the first 500 ewes in lowland flocks and the first 1000 ewes on holdings in a designated less favoured area. Half the premium was paid on ewes above these limits. A political agreement was reached by ministers on the 21 May 1992 on the reform of the Common Agricultural Policy, which will have far reaching effects on all sectors of the agricultural industry. In particular sheep reforms were limited to the establishment of an individual producer limit on the number of ewes which were eligible for premium based on numbers in a reference year which at the time of writing had still to be decided. Furthermore, the amount paid will be reduced by a 1% amount to create a national reserve which has to be set aside for the provision of ewe premium rights to new entrants into the industry. The annual ewe premium is paid in three instalments based on a

Table 3.2 Annual ewe premium payments (ECU/ewe). (Source: EC Commission)

	Sheep Marketing Year			
	1988	1989	1990	1991
Italy	18.9	18.6	23.8	20.4
Greece	18.9	18.6	23.8	20.4
France	18.9	18.6	23.8	20.4
Belgium	19.6	19.0	23.8	20.4
Luxembourg	19.6	19.0	23.8	20.4
Denmark	19.6	19.0	23.8	20.4
Germany	19.6	19.0	23.8	20.4
Netherlands	19.6	19.0	23.8	20.4
Irish Republic	21.0	21.8	27.5	25.8
Great Britain	9.1	10.3	14.1	16.6
Northern Ireland	18.0	19.0	27.5	25.8
Spain	15.3	13.0	16.7	20.4
Portugal	15.3	13.0	16.7	20.4

1 ECU = £0.78 at 1991 value.

forecast of the representative price for the marketing year in question. An additional special ewe premium is also paid to producers designated in less favoured areas from 1991. This amount is paid with the first instalment of the annual ewe premium.

Trade with non-EC countries
An important element of the regime involves trade with non-EC countries and is most detailed concerning imports. Voluntary Restraint Agreements (VRA) were agreed at the beginning of the regime with the principal supplying countries, the most important of which is New Zealand. The VRAs which were in force at the beginning of the 1991 marketing year are presented in Table 3.3. The large amounts allowed from New Zealand cover the import of frozen lamb to the UK which accounted for over 74% of the total EC sheepmeat imports in 1989. A number of countries have not negotiated VRAs and, on the basis of their traditional trade, they are allocated import quotas on an annual basis. Chile and Greenland are the most important countries which use annual quotas to sell lambs on the EC market. The EC signed associated agreements with Czechoslovakia,

Table 3.3 Voluntary restraint agreements, 1991 (t of carcase equivalent). (Source: MLC, 1992a)

	Sheepmeat		Live sheep
	Frozen	Fresh/Chilled	
Australia	14 500	3 000	
New Zealand	195 500	10 500	
Argentina	17 400	1 600	
Uruguay	2 600	2 600	
Bulgaria	1 250		2 000
Czechoslovakia		800	
Hungary		1 150	10 050
Poland		200	6 000
Iceland	540	60	
Austria			300
Romania		75	475
Yugoslavia		4 800	200

Poland and Hungary in October 1991 which allowed them to export a limited amount of sheepmeat and live sheep into the community at a reduced levy, in addition to their VRA quotas. The tonnage will be increased from 1992 to 1996.

Trade
The community is a net importer of sheepmeat, being approximately 85% self-sufficient. The deficit is made up mainly by imports of frozen lamb into the UK from New Zealand. Germany, Greece and Italy also import significant quantities of fresh/chilled and frozen sheepmeat from third countries, notably Argentina, Australia and eastern Europe. Italy is the major importer of live sheep most of which come from east European countries.

The major trade flows of sheepmeat in the community are shown in Table 3.4. Live sheep have been converted to a carcase equivalent and combined with the total for carcase meat. It can be seen that there is a considerable amount of intra-community trade and that over and above this only relatively small quantities of sheepmeat are sent to countries outside the community.

Although wool production in 1990 was 154 million kg in the EC, the volume of imports was three times greater. About half the production

Table 3.4 Major trade flows of sheepmeat in EC, 1991 (000 t). (Source: from MLC, 1992c)

Country	Total imports 1991	Origin				Others	
		New Zealand	Netherlands	Irish Republic	United Kingdom	E.E.C	Third countries
Belgium and Luxembourg	27.6				9.5	12.6	5.5
France	166.7		11.7	56.1	65.0	32.7	1.2
Greece	16.0	10.4				1.0	4.6
Italy	66.1	6.2				13	23.4
UK	104.9	93.7		1.7			9.5
Germany	35.2	20			2.1	1.9	11.2
Spain	32.9	6.3			5.3	18.0	1.0

was exported, leaving a net use of 506 million kg which represents 13% self-sufficiency in wool.

Production in the United Kingdom

Statistics on the UK industry are available from census data collected in June and December each year. A higher sheep population is recorded in June since all flocks will have lambed by June and only a small proportion of the lambs will have been sold. The December census figures, which provide the most reliable estimates of breeding ewe numbers, are summarized over a twelve year period in Fig. 3.1. Breeding ewe numbers have risen to an all time high in December 1992 with the latest estimate indicating a population of over twenty million breeding ewes.

Productivity from this large ewe population is varied and depends on breed, locality and the system of production under which they are kept. Average levels of production per ewe in 1989 were 19.6 kg of carcase meat, 1.8 kg of wool and 1.3 kg of sheepskin (FAO, 1991), but these averages conceal such a wide variation that they can only be used as a general guide.

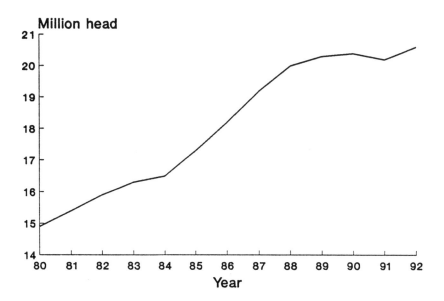

Fig. 3.1 United Kingdom breeding ewe population. (Source: MAFF)

The list of breeds and crossbreds available throughout the UK is extensive. In the latest edition of *British Sheep*, details from sixty-four societies for purebred sheep and eleven for crossbred sheep are presented (National Sheep Association, 1992). The crossbred sheep societies included in this publication are only the major organizations which are involved in some kind of co-operative marketing. In addition to these eleven, there is a long list of different crossbred types. Over 300 different crossbred ewes were reported in an MLC survey conducted in 1987 (MLC, 1988b). Further aspects of this survey are discussed and a more detailed description of the British sheep industry structure given in Chapter 7.

It is important to note here that 45% of the total breeding ewe population is located in hill areas, 17% in upland areas and 38% in the lowlands. Production in these three sectors will be discussed in more detail in later chapters.

The latest detailed UK census data available is for June 1991. This shows that 93 943 farms kept sheep and 89 974 farms kept breeding ewes, equivalent to an average flock size of 461 sheep and 226 ewes respectively. The expansion of breeding ewe numbers in recent years has arisen not only through increased flock size but also through an increase in the total number of flocks. Census data for England and Wales illustrates this point (Table 3.5).

Slaughterings from the 20.6 million ewes mated in 1990 amounted to 15.9 million lambs in the 1991–2 marketing year plus 1.6 million ewes and rams.

As a result of the varied nature of production, lamb supplies in the UK are seasonal. The monthly pattern of slaughterings is illustrated in Fig. 3.2. Typically, production in the early months of the year is from the previous year's lamb crop which is supplemented during late March/April by new season lamb from early lambing flocks.

Table 3.5 Changes in flock numbers and size in England and Wales 1980–91. (Source: MAFF)

	1980	1985	1991
Number of holdings with breeding ewes	56 441	59 600	64 000
Average number of breeding ewes per flock	185	198	223

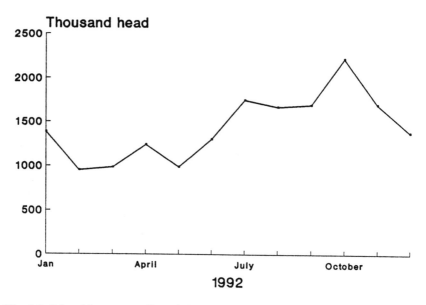

Fig. 3.2 Monthly seasonality of slaughterings. (Source: MAFF)

Production increases during June and July as many lowland flocks sell lambs from grass, and rises to a peak in September and October when upland and hill flocks market large numbers of lambs and the remainder of the lowland lambs produced at grass are also sold. Production declines to the end of the year with finished store lambs coming on to the market. Prices of finished lambs reflect these production levels, reaching a peak in early spring and then falling until September. The pattern of average market prices for 1992 is shown in Fig. 3.3.

The average market prices within any given month mask considerable variations which are attributable to the effects of live weight and region. When the overall range in weights (17–52 kg) is subdivided into more important weight bands it is noticeable that weights below 45 kg receive the highest price per kilogram and that there is a general tendency for price per kilogram to decline as weight increases (Table 3.6). Lighter lambs also follow this pattern, apart from during the spring period when light milk-fed lambs are in high demand for the Easter market. The price pattern within any one weight range over the year is similar and follows the trend illustrated in Fig. 3.3.

Regional price differences can also be found (Table 3.7) but these are less marked than variation due to carcase weight. The lower price per kilogram received for lambs marketed in Scotland is the most

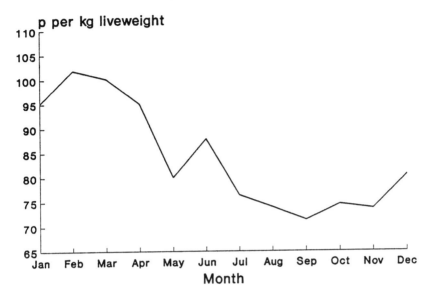

Fig. 3.3 Seasonal price variation. (Source: MLC, 1992b)

notable regional difference which partly reflects the large carcases produced. If these figures were adjusted for the effects of lamb weight, it is quite likely that regional differences would disappear.

An important point concerning the actual marketing of lambs is the high proportion of the annual lamb crop which is sold through the live auction market system. In 1992 over 70% of the lamb crop was marketed in this way.

In addition to slaughter lamb marketings, there is a large trade in lambs for further fattening, store lambs, and for breeding stock. Store lamb prices averaged £27.51 per head for lowland lambs and £21.42 per head for hill lambs in 1991. Average breeding stock prices for the same year ranged from £39 for ewe lambs to £54 for two-year-old lowland crossbreds. Ewes drafted from hill flocks to upland areas averaged £16, whill cull ewe prices varied seasonally and tended to follow the lamb price rather than the availability of cull ewes.

Industry statistics at all levels provide producers with the necessary information to organize and plan their sheep enterprises efficiently and in Britain the MLC Economics department is dedicated to the collection, interpretation and dissemination of data from the livestock industry. The main medium for dissemination is the written word, with regular weekly, monthly and yearly market reports and summaries for the main species. Sheep producers have access to average

Planned Sheep Production

Table 3.6 Variation in auction lamb prices in Great Britain by weight and month of sale in 1992 (p/kg lw). (Source: MLC, 1992b)

	Superlight (17.0–25.4 kg)	Light (25.5–32.0 kg)	Standard (32.1–39.0 kg)	Medium (39.1–45.5 kg)	Heavy (45.6–52.0 kg)	Others (Over 52 kg)
Jan	95.1	98.3	104.6	105.5	99.2	87.9
Feb	90.5	95.5	101.8	102.7	96.7	87.5
Mar	118.0	120.9	117.8	113.4	106.7	87.2
Apr	110.5	110.0	109.7	106.8	100.3	93.7
May	90.7	93.1	92.6	91.0	88.4	80.5
Jun	85.5	87.6	88.8	86.5	82.4	74.7
Jul	82.2	76.9	76.7	76.0	71.8	63.4
Aug	81.3	75.1	73.7	74.0	70.3	62.6
Sep	77.2	72.8	71.0	71.3	67.7	61.5
Oct	81.2	76.0	73.6	74.1	69.5	62.4
Nov	81.4	74.7	74.0	73.3	67.0	59.2
Dec	95.9	83.4	80.8	79.7	72.4	64.7

Table 3.7 Price per kg liveweight of finished lambs by region and month of sale in 1992 (p/kg lw). (Source: MLC, 1992b)

	Great Britain	England	Wales	Scotland
Jan	95.2	95.0	93.6	97.7
Feb	101.9	102.1	101.1	102.0
Mar	100.2	100.8	100.9	97.9
Apr	95.1	96.1	100.9	85.0
May	90.0	90.1	91.5	82.8
Jun	87.9	87.8	88.5	86.9
Jul	76.4	76.6	76.4	75.3
Aug	74.0	74.5	73.4	73.2
Sep	71.4	72.1	71.1	70.0
Oct	74.6	74.8	74.8	73.8
Nov	73.7	73.7	74.7	72.1
Dec	80.5	80.3	82.7	78.4

market prices and marketing levels, and regular in-depth evaluations of the sheep industry.

Section 2
Resources

The production of a successful plan for a sheep enterprise demands an understanding of the resources available to the flockmaster and an appreciation of the relationships between them. It is important that each resource is defined and the ways that it can be manipulated fully explored.

Three important resources can be identified: the animals themselves, the feed supplies and the associated fixed resources such as land, labour and capital. This section is devoted to the detailed consideration of each resource available to the sheep producer, and in conclusion explores their exploitation through industry structures. Attention has been confined to those aspects of production which have practical relevance and a potential application for commercial sheep producers.

4 Animal Resources

Breeding ewes

Observable differences in lamb production within similar types of production system in British flocks are mainly due to the varieties of breeding ewe involved and the differing standards of management. Technical innovations in reproductive physiology, such as out of season breeding, which can offer significant increases in ewe productivity are rarely adopted successfully by practical farmers and will not, therefore, be discussed in detail here. Concurrent with research interest in all the year round lambing systems was an increasing understanding of the principles of ewe nutrition which has been widely influential in the industry. In fact improved understanding of the principles of ewe nutrition coupled with an increasing awareness of the between breed variation existing amongst the British ewe population has brought about significant improvements in ewe productivity in recent years.

Maternal performance

While it is probably true to say that correct feeding of the ewe is the key to profitability regardless of the end-product or the environment in which she is kept, the genetic make-up of the ewe must also be suited to the demands made upon her. Some consideration of ewe genotypes and the variation between them is therefore essential for a complete treatment of planned sheep production.

Inevitably, nutrition and performance are interlinked. Reliable comparative performance data between breeds and crosses involves carefully controlled experimentation to ensure that all environmental influences on ewe performance are equal. Under British conditions these types of comparison are virtually impossible. Valid comparisons can only be made between sheep which have been born on the farm where they are observed. With the stratified structure of the British industry containing a large number of crossbred breeding ewes, this can be very expensive. Small scale experimentation does yield some useful comparative data between breeds but no major source of comparative data other than that collected from national recording schemes is available. These data have to be regarded with some caution as there are wide differences in management levels between the flocks from which they are drawn. However, in the absence of scientifically sound comparisons of ewe genotypes they form the most reliable source of independent estimates of performance.

Maternal characteristics
In whatever system of production or environment sheep are kept, ewes will be valued for one or more particular characteristics which may be directly related to the main product of the enterprise or may contribute indirectly to its success. Milk production is a good example of a maternal character which can be directly related to the productivity of the enterprise or related indirectly through its contribution to lamb growth rates. In France, milk production is directly relevant to certain milking breeds such as the Lacaune while for other breeds kept for meat production its value is directed towards good lamb growth rates. Under British conditions the latter is almost always the case.

The most important maternal character is undoubtedly the number of lambs sold per ewe. This in turn is the result of a number of related features, starting with fertility, ovulation rate, litter size, lamb survival, and milking and mothering ability. These are summarized, under commercial conditions, in terms of the proportion of barren ewes, the litter size and the number of lambs reared. The observed variation between the more common crossbred ewes found in Britain is small. The figures in Table 4.1 are averages taken over a number of years and involving several thousand ewe records, and as such can only be a guide to the potential of each genotype. Similar data for purebred ewes maintained under upland conditions shows slightly more variation (Table 4.2).

Guidance on the potential of each breed and cross can be obtained from recorded flocks. Within any one breed or cross there is considerable variation, probably as a direct result of management, and the higher levels of maternal performance observed among these flocks represent the potential of the genotype concerned. This within breed variation can be illustrated by a comparison between the top third flocks and average flocks (Table 4.3). Top third flocks are identified on the basis of gross margin per hectare and while that type

Table 4.1 Performance of common crossbred ewes in recorded lowland flocks in 1989. (Source: MLC, 1990)

	Per 100 ewes mated			Gross margin	
	Lambs born	Lambs reared	Overall stocking rate (ewes/ha)	£ Per ewe	£ Per ha
Bluefaced Leicester × Swaledale	171	164	13.2	35.40	467
Bluefaced Leicester × Scottish Blackface	157	151	10.1	40.00	404
Bluefaced Leicester × Welsh Mountain	158	147	12.9	35.20	454
Border Leicester × North Country Cheviot	151	143	11.7	36.70	429
Border Leicester × Welsh Mountain	145	138	13.9	34.90	485

Table 4.2 Performance of common purebred ewes in recorded upland flocks. (Source: MLC, 1979)

	Per 100 ewes mated			Lambs born per ewe lambing
	Lambs born alive	Lambs born dead	Lambs reared	
Beulah Speckle Face	129	8	119	1.38
Clun Forest	141	9	131	1.52
Scottish Blackface	130	9	120	1.40
Swaledale	131	8	121	1.41
Welsh Mountain	115	6	106	1.23

of comparison is not ideal for considering ewe performance characteristics it does serve to illustrate the likely variation. The sample of flocks from which the data presented in Table 4.3 was taken is different from the one used in Table 4.1. The variation within breeds is considerably greater than that between breeds and there is probably greater scope for increased ewe output within the flock through improved management than through breed substitution.

In addition to the maternal characteristics already discussed, others are of some importance. Ewe mature size is relevant to the number of ewes which can be supported on a given area and also to the potential carcase weights which can be produced from the flock, and these aspects will be covered at greater length later. Duration of the breeding season is an important characteristic in many situations. The extended season of the Dorset Horn and Poll Dorset is of considerable

Table 4.3 Performance of common crossbred ewes in average and top third recorded lowland flocks. (Source: MLC, 1990)

	Per 100 ewes mated			
	Empty	Lambs born alive	Lambs born dead	Lambs reared
Border Leicester × Scottish Blackface	5	163	11	153
(Scottish Halfbred)	**3**	**179**	**9**	**168**
Border Leicester × North Country Cheviot	5	159	12	150
(Greyface)	**3**	**179**	**16**	**165**
Border Leicester × Welsh Mountain	4	141	11	135
(Welsh Halfbred)	**3**	**158**	**15**	**147**
Bluefaced Leicester × Swaledale	5	167	9	160
(Mule)	**4**	**173**	**9**	**166**
Bluefaced Leicester × Scottish Blackface	6	157	7	151
(Scotch Mule)	**6**	**159**	**8**	**154**

Top third averages in bold type.

interest under British conditions for those production systems which involve out of season lambing in autumn and also for the small group of producers who follow an all the year round intensive system of management. Unfortunately, litter size is depressed in autumn and, therefore, more prolific Finnish Landrace crosses with the Dorset Horn have been developed to meet the requirements of systems of this type.

Wool yield and quality is, of course, an important characteristic but under British conditions it is of little economic consequence to the producer and is therefore often ignored. The reverse is true in wool producing areas of the world where considerable efforts are made to improve wool yield and quality.

Breed substitution and crossbreeding
Armed with detailed information on different breeds or crosses, flockmasters have the possibility of improving the profitability of their flock by breed substitution. Such a decision cannot be taken lightly as it may involve considerable cost outlay and a reorientation of management to make optimum use of the new animals' genetic potential. A most dramatic example of this type of breed substitution occurred

in British dairy herds during the late 1950s and 60s when the Friesian took over as the major dairy breed on the strength of its superior milk yield and was then in turn superseded during the 1970s by the North American Holstein. In the sheep industry, the Suffolk breed replaced the Oxford Down as the major terminal sire in the 1960s when large lambs, suitable for folding on roots and finishing at very heavy weights over the winter, were no longer appropriate. The Mule has emerged as the dominant type of lowland crossbred ewe in recent years. In 1971 there were estimated to be 311 000 Mules in Britain. By 1987 this had risen to 3.2 million, the most numerous ewe type in the country, and accounted for 17% of all ewes mated (MLC, 1988).

There are two basic requirements for successful breed substitution. Firstly, an accurate monitoring system for breed performance must be available in order to provide information upon which objective decisions can be based. Secondly, there must not be any appreciable genotype × environment interaction in the characters being considered for breed substitution or else the apparent superiority of the new breed in its own environment may not be transferred to the new environment. The most common misuse of breed substitution occurs when a breed is transported from its country of origin to another where climatic, nutritional or disease conditions may result in poorer performance.

Improved productivity can be achieved in sheep flocks by planned crossbreeding. Combining the genes of two or more separate breeds in a regular programme can lead to improvements in performance due to the combination of desirable traits from the different parent breeds in a useful mix. The system of early lamb production referred to earlier combines the prolificacy of the Finnish Landrace with the extended breeding season of the Dorset Horn to advantage. When mated to one of the smaller terminal sire breeds the resultant females produce well finished carcases for the Easter lamb trade. A similar system is operated in Spain by one private company, utilizing native breeds crossed with the Romanov to produce ewes which when mated to Île de France rams produce lambs for slaughter.

As well as on an individual farm basis, crossbreeding can be utilized on a national scale. A large part of the British sheep industry is concerned with the production and utilization of crossbreds but consideration of these aspects is left until Chapter 7.

Crossbreeding can also be used to improve the expected level of performance in particular traits by utilizing hybrid vigour ('heterosis'). Under commercial conditions it is difficult to demonstrate the existence of hybrid vigour. However, Nitter (1978) has reviewed its extent under experimental conditions and this indicates that lamb survival demonstrates a high degree of hybrid vigour, lamb weight for age a moderate level and reproductive traits a low level when the effect of crossing two purebreds is looked at. When considering the performance of crossbred ewes, however, the improvement in fertility due to heterosis is much higher. These effects no doubt contribute to the continuing use of the stratified crossbreeding structure found in Britain.

Enhancing maternal performance

Increased levels of reproductive performance are made possible by shortening the interval between pregnancies using non-nutritional management techniques such as early weaning, oestrus synchronization and stimulation by progesterone analogues, or through enhanced litter size by treatment with pregnant mare's serum gonadotrophin (PMSG). These techniques are appropriate for the more intensive systems of production where nutrition is unrestricted and there is little seasonal limitation of herbage growth and availability. A number of examples of frequent lambing systems utilize these techniques (Tempest, 1983), but they have not been widely applied in practice.

Synchronized breeding in the normal mating season is practised by a number of commercial producers for the benefits afforded by better management and improved lamb marketing. Progestogen impregnated intra-vaginal sponges are a cheap and practical means of synchronizing ewes. Sponges are placed in the vagina for 12–16 days and at sponge withdrawal an injection of 500 international units of PMSG ensures a high oestrus response and enhanced litter size. One problem with PMSG, however, is the variable litter size response to a given dose.

Body condition scoring

The level of body condition at mating has been shown to have a direct bearing on ovulation and conception rate. Although everyone working with sheep has a personal method of assessing body condition, descriptions of condition tend to be imprecise since they use equivocal phrases such as 'poor', 'fairly good' or 'moderate store'. What is considered to be 'forward store' by someone accustomed to working with lowland sheep might be termed 'very good' by someone more familiar with hill stock. A standardized system of body condition scoring was therefore developed from an Australian method by the

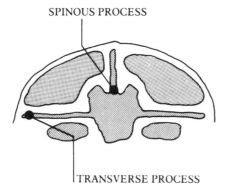

SPINOUS PROCESS

TRANSVERSE PROCESS

Fig. 4.1 Cross section through lumbar region

Hill Farming Research Organisation (HFRO) to overcome such difficulties (Russel, Doney & Gunn, 1969). It is based on a six-point scale, from 0 to 5, and to a half-point accuracy.

Condition is assessed by finger pressure along the top and sides of the backbone in the loin area immediately behind the last rib and above the kidneys. A cross section through this area is presented in Fig. 4.1 to illustrate the important handling points which are assessed in the following order:

(1) The sharpness or roundness of the spinous processes of the lumbar vertebrae (the bony points rising upwards from the back).
(2) The prominence and degree of cover of the transverse processes of the vertebrae (the bone protruding from each side of the backbone).
(3) The extent of muscular and fatty tissues underneath the transverse processes (judged by the ease with which the fingers pass under the ends of the bones).
(4) The fullness and fat cover of the eye muscle (judged by pressing between the spinous and transverse processes).

On the basis of the handling characteristics of the ewe, a score is awarded according to the scale given in Table 4.4. In practice, the extreme points of the scale (score 0 and score 5) are rarely used and most ewes score between 1½ and 4½. It must be emphasized that the technique is subjective and occasions arise where animals do not fit exactly into these neat categories.

Body condition scoring is easy both to learn and to use and does not

Table 4.4 Condition scores. (Source: Russel, Doney & Gunn, 1969)

Condition score	Handling characteristics
0	Extremely emaciated and on the point of death. It is not possible to detect any muscular or fatty tissue between the skin and the bone.
1	The spinous processes are prominent and sharp; the transverse processes are also sharp, the fingers pass easily under the ends, and it is possible to feel between each process; the loin muscles are shallow with no fat cover.
2	The spinous processes are prominent but smooth, individual processes can be felt only as fine corrugations; the transverse processes are smooth and rounder, and it is possible to pass the fingers under the ends with a little pressure; the loin muscles are of moderate depth, but have little fat cover.
3	The spinous processes have only a small elevation, are smooth and rounded, and individual bones can be felt only with pressure; the transverse processes are smooth and well covered, and firm pressure is required to feel over the ends; the loin muscles are full, and have a moderate degree of fat cover.
4	The spinous processes can just be detected with pressure as a hard line; the ends of the transverse processes cannot be felt; the loin muscles are full and have a thick covering of fat.
5	The spinous processes cannot be detected even with firm pressure; there is a depression between the layers of fat where the spinous processes would normally be felt; the transverse processes cannot be detected; the loin muscles are very full with very thick fat cover.

require any equipment. It overcomes the problems of differences in size and skeletal shape of ewes which can affect bodyweights and it can be used in situations where bodyweights are difficult to interpret, e.g. in pregnant ewes.

In general, the better the condition at mating, the higher is the ovulation rate and the higher the lambing percentage. The aim should be to get ewes in condition score 3 ½ at mating, though achieving this is no guarantee of a good lamb crop. Sound sheep husbandry is required throughout pregnancy and early lactation to cash in on good body condition at mating.

The close relationship between condition at mating and lambing percentage in recorded flocks is shown in Table 4.5. These figures suggest that condition score 3 ½ at mating is needed to achieve the best lambing results. Experience has shown that in the majority of flocks scores range from 1 ½ to 4 and that specific groups of ewes would benefit from an improvement in condition before mating. Although poor conception rates can be expected from both overfat and overthin ewes, MLC records indicate that the latter is the more common problem: 18% of lowland ewes have condition scores of 2 or less and 4% have scores of 4 ½ to 5 at mating. Scoring at the beginning of mating demonstrates the importance of good body condition on subsequent performance, but at this stage it only reflects recent nutrition and it is too late to effect improvement.

In order to allow sufficient time for improvement, flocks should be scored six to eight weeks before the rams are turned out since body condition can be markedly influenced by management at this time. Positive action is needed to reduce the number of ewes in poor condition six weeks before mating, and it follows that they must be weaned in good time. Those scoring 2 ½ can normally be expected to

Table 4.5 Lambing percentages for ewes in various body conditions at mating. (Source: MLC, 1988a)

	1	1 ½	2	2 ½	3	3 ½	4
				Body condition score at mating			
				Lambs born per 100 ewes to ram			
Hill ewes							
Scottish Blackface		79			162		
Hill Gritstone			75	103	119	109	
Welsh Mountain	60	65	105	116	123		
Swaledale		78	133	140	156		
Lowland							
Gritstone (lowland)				132	154	173	
Masham				167	181	215	
Mule			149	166	178	194	192
Greyface			147	163	176	189	184
Welsh Halfbred		126	139	150	164	172	
Scottish Halfbred			148	170	183	217	202

reach a score of 3 by tupping, but ewes scoring 2 or below require special treatment. They should be drawn out of the flock and given the best available grazing. Alternatively, the stocking rate can be reduced and supplementary concentrate feed provided if necessary. Weaned ewes respond quickly to increased feeding and should easily achieve the required mating condition score of 3 within six to eight weeks. A sample of the ewes receiving preferential treatment should be scored after three weeks to check that the necessary improvement is being made. Results of an MLC trial demonstrate that significant improvements in lambing performance can be achieved through condition scoring six weeks prior to mating and then taking remedial action (Table 4.6).

These results emphasize the benefits of condition scoring in advance of mating in order that some positive course of action may be taken. Condition scoring is an essential planning tool which is widely adopted under British conditions, and it can be used at all times of the sheep year. Anyone undertaking the assessment of body condition for the first time is advised to seek help or advice.

Ewe nutrition

The profitability of any sheep enterprise is to a large extent dependent on meeting the nutritional requirements of the ewe. These requirements will vary according to a wide range of circumstances such as the type of ewe, the production system and the stage in the production cycle. It is important, therefore, to understand how these factors inter-

Table 4.6 Comparison of flock conditions scored six weeks before mating and (a) treated (b) not treated. (Source: Pollott & Kilkenny, 1976a)

	(a) Treated flocks			(b) Untreated flocks		
	Poor ewes	Rest of flock	Difference	Poor ewes	Rest of flock	Difference
Average condition score six weeks before mating	1.7	3.0	1.3	1.7	2.9	1.2
Average condition at mating	2.8	3.2	0.4	2.3	3.0	0.7
Lambs born per 100 ewes to ram	147	160	13	135	160	25

relate to achieve the required levels of performance. Lower levels of performance are accepted in hill areas because of harsh climatic conditions and poor quality grazings, but body reserves can be replenished when forage is in good supply. Under more intensive conditions the ewe may be expected to perform at her peak throughout the year. Ewe feeding must therefore be designed to provide enough nutrients at all stages of the production cycle.

It is beyond the scope of this book to provide diets for all sheep in all conditions. Such a task is best dealt with using a computer model (see, for example, France, Neal & Pollott, 1982) which can cope with a wide variety of different circumstances. A much more exhaustive treatment of the subject can be found in *Feeding the Ewe* (MLC, 1988a).

In this section the different stages of the production cycle are considered in turn and an example ration given. Target body condition scores will also be used as a guide to correct feeding.

Weaning to mating
The time between weaning and mating can be a critical period during which the success of the whole enterprise is determined. Ewes should be prepared for mating during this period so that they are in the optimum condition for mating and thus produce the required number of ova. Overfatness at mating can lead to barrenness and metabolic problems at lambing, while poor condition at mating can result in barrenness and low lambing percentages.

One method for using condition scoring as a means of assessing the requirements of the ewe before mating has already been described. The subject of 'flushing' ewes before mating has received considerable attention from research workers over the years (see Cockrem, 1979; Rhind, 1992) and their conclusions have not always been clear. Some confusion has arisen in the past due to the use of body weight as an indication of nutritional status. Also the importance of the starting condition of the animal was not always appreciated and foetal loss may have confused some results. It would appear that ovulation rate can be affected by the level of energy intake immediately prior to mating, but only over an intermediate range of condition scores. This range varies with the type of ewe and the extent of the variation is difficult to predict accurately. Other considerations such as appetite may also be factors in the response to 'flushing'. It is clear, however, that ovulation rate improves with condition at mating up to the level where problems occur from overfatness.

Example ration

(1) Ewes required to gain one condition score over the eight weeks before mating: 2.4 kg of hay per ewe per day.
(2) Ewes required to maintain condition over the weeks prior to mating: 1.5 kg of hay per ewe per day.

N.B. In this chapter all example rations have been calculated for a 70 kg twin-bearing ewe fed on good quality hay and a 16% crude protein concentrate.

Early pregnancy
Although a great deal of work looking at the affects of premating treatment on lambing performance has been carried out, it is only recently that attention has been turned to the immediate post-mating period. The first four weeks of pregnancy are an important phase in foetal development. During the first two weeks after mating the developing embryo is not attached to the uterus and receives its nourishment by direct absorption from its fluid environment. Implantation of the embryo takes place during the third week after mating. The placenta then grows rapidly and the developing foetus becomes increasingly dependent on the placenta for its supply of nutrients from the ewe.

Since an abrupt change in plane of nutrition during the first four weeks of gestation can adversely affect the survival and proper development of the embryo, it is recommended that the ewe should be maintained on the mating ration for the first four weeks of pregnancy. Thus lowland ewes should continue to graze the better pastures used for mating and, since this period normally coincides with a reduction in the growth and quality of herbage, the stocking rates may need adjustment to maintain the plane of nutrition. Hill ewes mated in-bye or on improved pasture should continue to graze there for as long as possible. Before they return permanently to the hill, a few days of free access between the improved pasture and hill grazings will smooth the transition and avoid a sudden change in the level of nutrition.

Example ration
1.5 kg of hay per ewe per day.

Mid-pregnancy

During the second and third months of pregnancy the placenta, the uterus and the foetuses all undergo some increase in weight. The foetuses, by now well attached to the uterus of the ewe, grow quite slowly at this stage (Fig. 4.2). By the end of the third month of pregnancy the placenta is fully developed but the foetus itself is only about 15% of its weight at birth which can be anything from 1 kg to 2.5 kg depending on ewe size and litter size.

With mature ewes which were in the correct body condition at mating (body score 3–3½), the aim in this period is to maintain apparent bodyweight with a reduction of about 0.5 units of body condition score. Loss of body condition greater than 0.75 units must be avoided if the birth weight and the survival chances of the lamb are not to be impaired. Care must be taken not to feed appreciably above these levels, however, since this can lead to overfat ewes which are much more susceptible to metabolic disorders such as pregnancy toxaemia in late pregnancy.

Example ration

Minimum level of intake 1.2 kg of hay per ewe per day.

Ewe lambs in lowland flocks, two year old ewes in hill flocks and mature ewes which were mated in poor body condition should be allowed to make a steady gain in weight during this period amounting to about one body score. In addition ewe lambs in lowland flocks should be allowed to grow and gain weight during this period.

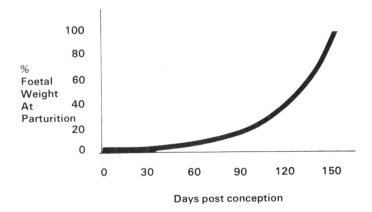

Fig. 4.2 Foetal growth. (Source: MLC, 1988a)

Example ration
1.8 kg of hay per ewe per day.

Recent advances in the use of real-time medical ultrasound equipment have enabled the sheep producer to estimate accurately the number of foetuses that a ewe is carrying at about the eighth week of gestation. In the hands of an experienced operator these scanning machines can be used to see the exact number of lambs being carried with up to almost 100% accuracy. Although with the exception of being able to cull barren ewes there is little advantage in knowing the litter size at such an early stage, in later pregnancy this information can be vital.

Late pregnancy
By the fourteenth week of pregnancy the placenta is well developed and the major tissues and organs of the foetuses have been formed, but the foetuses are still relatively small and about 70% of foetal growth will take place during the final six weeks of pregnancy (Fig. 4.2). The aim during this period is to achieve vigorous lambs of satisfactory birth weight. Additionally, provision must be made for lactation since most of the secretory tissue in the ewe's udder is laid down during this period. At lambing the adequately fed mature ewe carrying twins should have increased in gross weight by about 18% although this may represent a body score of only 2 to 2½.

The objective of rationing during this period is to gradually increase the level of feeding over the last eight weeks to meet the growing demands of the foetuses. Since appetite can be expected to decline in the last two to three weeks of pregnancy, particularly with ewes carrying multiple foetuses, the diet must gradually be concentrated. This is normally achieved in practice by introducing a concentrate at about six to eight weeks before lambing and then gradually increasing the daily allowance. Failure to feed adequately during this critical period can result in pregnancy toxaemia in the ewe, small weak lambs at birth and reduced milk yields during lactation.

Research has highlighted the importance of correct protein intakes at this stage in pregnancy (see Robinson, 1990). In sheep the dietary protein is largely broken down, or degraded, to ammonia by micro-organisms in the rumen. The extent of this breakdown, however, varies with the protein source and the length of time the protein stays in the rumen. In general the proteins in oats, barley and roots are about 90% degraded, the proteins in maize, wheat, groundnut and grass about 77% degraded, the protein in soya bean meal about 55% degraded and the protein in fish meal only about 35% degraded. The ammonia produced from these dietary proteins is used by the micro-organisms in the rumen to build up their own body protein which subsequently becomes available to the host animal as microbial protein. Dietary protein which is not degraded passes through the rumen into the lower digestive tract and there becomes available as a source of protein to the sheep.

In mid pregnancy the protein requirements of the ewe for the growth of the foetuses, placenta and uterine fluids are relatively small and can be met by microbial protein, provided that the diet contains at least 8% crude protein in the dry matter. However, during the last four weeks of pregnancy and in early lactation the protein requirements of the ewe for foetal growth, colostrum production and to meet the high output of protein in the milk will be greater than the supply of microbial protein, and hence some dietary protein which has not been broken down in the rumen will be required. This is provided as undegraded protein. The diet at this time should therefore include a proportion of feeds of low degradability such as soya bean meal or fish meal. Where ewes are inadequately fed in early lactation, the provision of dietary protein supplements of low degradability (e.g. fish meal) allows the ewe to use her body fat reserves efficiently to enhance milk yield. Most multiple bearing ewes will require rations containing an undegradable protein source in order to meet their requirements and counter the effects of reduced appetite in the last three weeks of pregnancy.

Example ration

(1) Ewes kept indoors: six weeks before lambing 1.9 kg of hay per ewe per day, but introduce some concentrate to make the transition from an all forage diet easier.

(2) Ewes kept indoors: two weeks before lambing 1.6 kg of hay and 0.8 kg of concentrate containing a source of undegradable protein.

The use of an accurate foetal count in mid-pregnancy has already been described, and there are several benefits in being able to divide the ewes into groups of single, twin and triplet bearing ewes and feed them accordingly. A saving in feed may be possible due to more accurate rationing according to the ewes' foetal burden. A reduced incidence of pregnancy toxaemia should occur when the amount of feed is better matched to requirements. Lamb losses should be reduced due to the production of lambs of a viable size, i.e. smaller singles and larger triplets, and the ewes being in better condition. In addition, finding foster mothers for triplet lambs is a simpler task at the all too hectic lambing time.

White and Russel (1987) quoted a possible range in economic benefit of £2,50 in hill flocks to £4.75/ewe in intensive lowland flocks. For an initial outlay of about £0.75/ewe this seems to be an economic practice.

Early lactation
During the first six weeks of its life the lamb receives the major part of its nutrients from the ewe's milk and the aim of good feeding practice should be to maximize the amount of milk available to the lamb in this period. To some extent the basis of a good milk supply will have already been laid down during pregnancy. A ewe lambing down in good condition (body score 2 ½ to 3) will be able to cope with the birth process and the demands made upon it in early lactation better than a ewe in poor condition. Lambs suckling ewes in poor condition will eventually be able to compensate for the reduced milk supply by eating more grass, but this is an inefficient process.

The level of milk production from a ewe depends on several factors. The most influential is the number of lambs suckled (Table 4.7). Ewes suckling twins can produce 40% more milk than those suckling singles

Table 4.7 Potential milk yields (kg per day) of ewes in different environments. (Source: MLC, 1988a)

	Month of lactation		
	1st	2nd	3rd
Suckling twin lambs			
Lowland and improved upland	3.00	2.25	1.50
Hill	1.90	1.60	1.10
Suckling single lambs			
Lowland and improved upland	2.10	1.70	1.05
Hill	1.25	1.05	0.70

under exactly the same conditions. More vigorous lambs can also stimulate milk production. There are some breed effects on milk production although differences are small between breeds of a similar size. Within breed differences can be large. There is a steady rise in lactation yield from the first to third lactation which then levels off until the sixth lactation. The decline in yield after this point depends very much on the condition of the ewe, but with careful management milk yield can continue to be adequate.

Although voluntary food intake increases rapidly after lambing it will in most situations be difficult to meet the ewe's requirements during this period. Some loss of liveweight may be necessary in order to maintain a good milk supply, thus highlighting the reason why feeding 'for lactation' during pregnancy is important. Losses in the order of half a body score in the first six weeks of lactation can be tolerated without a significant reduction in milk yield. However, above this level milk yield may decline by around 15% for a loss in condition of one body score.

In order to keep bodyweight losses to a minimum it is important to feed high quality diets and to include in these some undegradable protein source. Intakes for different quality diets during the first weeks of lactation are shown in Fig. 4.3. In situations where the ewe is turned out to graze immediately after lambing, care must be taken to ensure that an adequate supply of good grass is available. If turnout occurs before the start of grass growth then a ration to meet the full requirements of the ewe must be fed.

Example ration
2 kg of hay and 0.75 kg of concentrate per ewe per day. The concentrate ration should contain an undegradable protein source.

Late lactation
After about the sixth week of lactation milk yield starts to decline, and soon afterwards the body condition of the ewe levels out. Provided that a good standard of feeding is maintained, some recovery in body condition from the second month of lactation onward can occur. If high lamb growth rates are to be maintained the lambs must have access to good quality grazing as their dependence on the ewe's milk begins to decline. If grazing is poor then the lamb and ewe will begin to compete for the available grass. Under such conditions it is worth

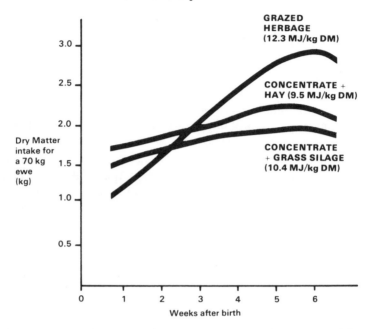

Fig. 4.3 Voluntary feed intakes in early lactation by ewes suckling twin lambs (metabolizable energy concentration of the complete diet shown in brackets). (Source: MLC, 1988a)

giving the lamb preferential treatment in the form of better grazing or concentrates fed in a creep system.

As the ewe's lactation begins to decline rapidly, access to good quality forage can lead to a further increase in body reserves. However, it is more usual, especially in hill conditions, to find that the grass quality is poor and that the ewes do not have a chance to recover body condition until after weaning.

A broader discussion of feeds and grazing has been left until Chapter 5.

Breeding rams

The ram is often forgotten as a major contributor to the success of the commercial flock. In terms of influence on the lamb crop produced each year, rams are significantly more important than individual ewes and, if ignored in the general care and management of the flock, can lead to disappointing levels of flock fertility. Most damage to stock rams arises during the ten months of the year when they are not in use, and usually through neglect.

Ram selection

There are no certainties when buying replacement stock rams but the more information that is available on the ram and his close relatives, the more likely is the ram to give satisfaction in terms of settling ewes and siring better than average lambs. Important aspects to consider when choosing a replacement ram are breed, fitness for work, performance information, conformation and the health status of the flock of origin.

Breed is important in the context of the product. In Britain the breed of terminal sire chosen can have a marked influence on lamb value, influencing carcase weight and sale date of the finished lamb. In wool producing countries it may have an important bearing on the wool yield of its progeny in the next generation.

The ram's fitness for work and conformation should be considered from the point of view of his function. Certainly, rams should be in good health and free from signs of infectious or contagious disease. The feet and legs must be sound if the ram is to mount ewes and successfully serve them, while good jaw conformation, with square flat incisor teeth biting on the dental pad, is vital. The ram's external genitalia should be well developed and free from any detectable abnormalities. Some detailed examination of the genitalia is necessary, with the ram sitting on his tail. The prepuce area should be checked for any ulceration and for free movement of the penis through the orifice of the prepuce. The penis can be checked when it is extracted. It should be free from inflammation and freely moveable. The scrotum must be handled carefully to ensure that the skin is supple and that there are no adhesions joining the skin to the testicles, which should be ovoid and large. Normally there should be two, but the absence of one does not mean that the ram is infertile. If it is used in a pedigree flock, however, it may pass on this trait. The testicles should be even in size and resilient to pressure. Two well defined tails of epididymis at the end of the testicles should be closely examined for it is here that the sperm will spend up to fourteen days maturing. There should be no lumps in this area.

Management of young rams

It is advisable to acquire young rams eight to ten weeks in advance of mating to allow time for them to settle down. On arrival at the farm the aim should be to integrate them slowly to avoid harassment by older rams. Handling with care and keeping stress to a minimum will be rewarded as stress can result in a reluctance and even an inability to work. Any injections should be administered as far in advance of mating as possible.

Young ram lambs should start mating at condition score 3 to 3 ½ as they can be expected to lose some condition during the mating period. Breeders normally rear their ram lambs on a high plane of nutrition to allow their full growth potential to be expressed, and wherever possible the diet provided by the breeder should be simulated. If this is not possible it must be remembered that the nutritive value of autumn grass can be low and that concentrate feeding may be desirable. Supplementary feeding will also encourage the ram to come to hand and facilitate regular inspection throughout its life, particularly during mating.

Under British conditions, ram lambs should not be run with more than thirty ewes and these should preferably be experienced ewes. It is advisable to raddle the ram so that his performance may be easily monitored. While concentrate feeding during mating, the raddle harness can be thoroughly checked and the ram examined for undue abrasion. Harness sores are stressful and should be avoided.

Routine health precautions are advisable, but before any action check with the breeder of the ram on the routine veterinary treatments already administered. Protection from clostridial disease and pasturella is certainly advisable. A foot-rot vaccine is also advisable if this is used in the flock, but not just before mating. Such vaccination does not, however, remove the obligation to routinely examine the feet or use a footbath subsequently.

Mature rams
At the end of the mating season the ram should be held in good condition for the rest of the year on clean grazing. To be fit, well and ready for use in the next season rams must receive regular attention and be maintained in good body condition. Libido and sperm production can be reduced by poor body condition, and regular condition scoring through the year is therefore essential. The aim is for the ram to be in body condition score 3 ½ to 4 by mating, and this may require some remedial action eight weeks prior to mating as in the management of breeding ewes.

A general examination of the ram to include conformation, general health and genitalia should also be made in advance of mating so that new ram requirements can be planned well in advance. The sexual ability of a ram will tend to decline from five years of age onwards, so elderly rams must be scrutinized regularly if they are not to let the flock down.

Artificial insemination

Despite a wealth of knowledge on the technique of semen collection and storage and the insemination of ewes, the use of artificial insemination (AI) in Britain is limited. This contrasts dramatically with the situation found in many other sheep producing countries which run extensive AI services for sheep producers. The techniques employed in AI are similar wherever a service is offered.

Semen may be collected routinely throughout the year from rams using a teaser ewe and an artificial vagina. Ram training time varies according to the age of the ram and the time of year. Rams under two years have significantly lower semen production and are less inclined to work than adult rams. About 10% of ram lambs cannot be trained to the collection routine.

The season of the year and frequency of collection influence sperm production, volume and concentrations (Table 4.8). Using these collection frequencies and current storage and insemination techniques, it is estimated that 95% of adult rams have a potential annual semen production in the range of 2500 to 5000 doses of deep-frozen semen or 6000 to 8000 doses of fresh chilled semen per ram. Compared to bulls and boars, ram semen has a low volume and high sperm concentration.

Assessment of semen quality involves examination for semen motility and the percentage of abnormal spermatazoa in the sample. By using a simple semen scoring system (ATB, 1989) it is possible to assess semen collections on-farm. A semen score is allocated to an ejaculate on the basis of its appearance, ranging from 0 (clear/watery)

Table 4.8 Seasonal semen characteristics from adult Suffolk rams. (Source: MLC, 1982)

	Ejaculate volume (ml)	Average sperm numbers per ejaculate (000 000)	Maximum weekly ejaculates
September–January	1.1	3.83	20
March–August	0.8	3.16	5

to 5 (thick cream). The scores indicate the approximate number of sperm per ml, provide a simple classification system for rams and, when combined with a motility assessment, provide a practical on-farm method of determining the suitability of semen for AI. Short term storage involves dilution with a heat treated diluent prepared from milk or egg yolk, antibiotics, sugars and cryoprotectants as necessary. Dilution is important on two counts: the increased use of semen from an individual ram and the provision of suitable nutrients for the spermatazoa. Semen can either be stored fresh at 15°C for use within 10–12 h or frozen at –196°C for use over several years.

The insemination technique involves oestrus synchronization to allow the insemination of a group of selected ewes at a predetermined time. At present the use of progestogen impregnated intravaginal sponges followed by an injection of PMSG appears to provide the best commercially available synchronization method. The most important points which influence conception rates are the number of inseminations, single or double, and whether the semen is fresh or frozen (Table 4.9). Single inseminations should be made 55–57 hours after injection of PMSG while 50 and 60 hours post injection is recommended for double inseminations.

The lower conception rates with frozen semen restrict the wider use of AI in the British industry. Recent research interest has centred on intra-uterine insemination with frozen semen, involving a minor surgical incision. This method offers increased conception rates to the levels associated with fresh semen at a double insemination.

AI must be carried out with the minimum of disturbance and suitable ewe handling facilities are necessary to minimize stress. Individuals need to be restrained to allow location of the cervix (the insemination site) with an illuminated vaginal speculum. Insemination rates of around 60 ewes per hour are possible.

Table 4.9 Anticipated conception rates. (Source: MLC, 1982)

Semen type	Insemination method	Conception rates%
Fresh diluted	Single	65
	Double	70
Frozen	Single	33
	Double	56
Frozen	Intra-uterine	70

Lamb growth and carcase characteristics

Liveweight growth
The maximum potential growth rate of a lamb is an inherited character which will reflect both the breed characteristics of its parents and their particular genetic merit. Under most commercial conditions, however, this is of little significance since the economics of production have a greater influence on growth than the actual genetic potential of the lamb. The main economic factors which determine lamb growth are the type of end product, the price of that product and the amount of feed that can be used in the most cost effective manner to produce it. In addition to these economic constraints, factors such as the sex of the lamb, its rearing status and the health of the flock also combine to influence actual growth.

The idealized pattern of lamb growth is usually considered to be a linear increase in weight from birth until the animal achieves half its adult weight. Growth rate then declines until it stops at maturity. The pattern of growth is basically determined by the intake of energy relative to liveweight in the early stages. Although it is nearly impossible to measure growth rate under ideal conditions, values of up to 600 g/day have been found in individual cases in Britain. Perhaps of more interest to commercial lamb producers is the relationship between stage of maturity and the body composition of the lamb, particularly with regard to the different components of the carcase and the effects of differing growth rates on this relationship.

Both the breed and the sex of the lamb appear to influence the pattern of development of the important carcase components when comparisons are made at equal weights. However, such differences largely disappear when the comparisons are made at the same proportion of adult weight. When environmental conditions allow a comparison to be made it also seems that heavier breeds tend to grow faster than lighter ones.

Breed effects on carcase composition
Where lamb carcase production is the primary aim of the enterprise, as is often the case in Britain, considerable interest is centred on the influence that different breeds can have on the end product. Breeds of ewe are generally fixed on any particular farm and thus interest is therefore confined mainly to the choice of terminal sire breeds.

A large scale breed comparison trial was carried out by MLC over a five year period to look at the growth and carcase characteristics of the

Table 4.10 Breeds used in the MLC ram breed comparison trial. (Source: Croston *et al.*, 1987)

	Breed weights (kg)
Border Leicester	94
Dorset Down	77
Hampshire Down	78
Île de France	78
North Country Cheviot	82
Oxford Down	100
Southdown	61
Suffolk	91
Texel	87
Wensleydale	101

more important terminal sire breeds and also to gain information on recent importations of Île de France and Texel sheep. Ten sire breeds were involved in a range of different production systems using three common types of ewe: draft Scottish Blackface, Border Leicester × North Country Cheviot and Bluefaced Leicester × Swaledale. Numbers used per breed and breed weights (discussed later in this chapter) are presented in Table 4.10. A fixed number of lambs from each ram were slaughtered at predetermined weights in order that the growth of the carcase and its constituents could be studied over a range of weights. Half the carcases were fully dissected to provide carcase data (see Kempster, Croston, Guy & Jones, 1987; Croston, Kempster, Guy & Jones, 1987). The important results as far as the commercial producer aiming to sell lambs off grass is concerned are presented in Table 4.11.

Lambs under British conditions are drawn for slaughter at a given level of finish and results were therefore compared at a constant level of subcutaneous fat cover equivalent to the midpoint of fat class 3 in the MLC sheep carcase classification scheme (see page 84). Carcase weight at a constant fat cover was found to increase linearly with increased breedweight and, because no differences were detected in daily liveweight gain between breeds, the average number of days to finishing also increased with breedweight (Fig. 4.4).

The most important finding was the absence of any real breed differences in terms of carcase composition, particularly percentage lean in the carcase, apart from with the Texel breed. The Texel was

Table 4.11 Breed means for growth and carcase characteristics compared at the same level of subcutaneous fat cover (11.9%). (Source: Kempster *et al.*, 1987)

	Carcase weight (kg)	Age at slaughter (days)	Conformation (15-point scale)	% lean
Border Leicester	19.8$_e$	208$_e$	7.1$_a$	54.6$_a$
Dorset Down	17.2$_b$	153$_{ab}$	8.4$_{bc}$	55.0$_a$
Hampshire Down	17.7$_b$	162$_{abc}$	8.2$_{bc}$	54.6$_a$
Île de France	18.4$_c$	172$_{bcd}$	7.2$_a$	54.2$_a$
North Country Cheviot	18.9$_d$	187$_d$	7.7$_{ab}$	54.7$_a$
Oxford Down	20.1$_{ef}$	190$_d$	7.8$_{ab}$	54.3$_a$
Southdown	16.3$_a$	148$_a$	8.3$_c$	55.1$_a$
Suffolk	19.6$_e$	176$_{cd}$	8.5$_{bc}$	54.6$_a$
Texel	19.5$_e$	182$_{cd}$	8.8$_c$	56.5$_b$
Wensleydale	20.6$_f$	224$_e$	7.2$_a$	55.2$_a$

Sire breed means with the same suffix do not differ significantly at the 5% level.

shown to have a superior lean percentage as a result of a better lean to bone ratio and a better ratio of subcutaneous fat to intermuscular fat. Results involving the Texel were similar to other research findings both from the Animal Breeding Research Organization (ABRO) and

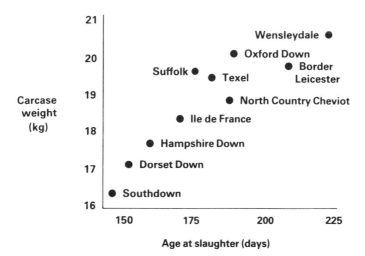

Fig. 4.4 Sire breed effects on growth and carcase weight. (Source: Kempster *et al.*, 1987)

Table 4.12 Age, carcase weight and conformation for Suffolk crosses at different fat classes. (Source: Kempster *et al.*, 1987)

	MLC fat class		
	2	3	4
Age at slaughter (days)	152	176	200
Carcase weight (kg)	17.5	19.6	21.7
Conformation scale (15-pt scale)	6.8	8.5	10.2

from Ireland, but the absolute superiority of the Texel over the other breeds was not so high as in the other trials.

Average carcase weights, fat levels and conformation scores are given in Table 4.12 for Suffolk-cross lambs at three fat classes, and no evidence was found to suggest that the other breeds grew in any other way. The general relationship between carcase weight and fat class is shown in Fig. 4.5. One of the main practical results of this trial was to demonstrate the relationship between potential mature weight of a particular breed or cross and its carcase weight at any given level of finish.

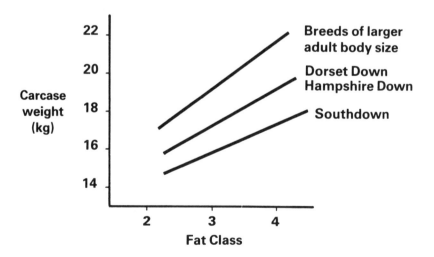

Fig. 4.5 General relationship between carcase weight and fat class. (Source: Kempster *et al.*, 1987)

Lamb nutrition

The provision of energy, protein, minerals and vitamins is necessary for healthy lamb growth and these may come from a range of sources including milk, cereals, grass and other vegetable matter. In turn, the availability of the required nutrients from these sources will depend on the physiological state of the rumen, the lamb's appetite, the digestibility of the food and the state of health of the lamb. The economics of different lamb production systems will ultimately determine how lambs are fed. In practice, lamb feeding is not always designed to maximize lamb growth rate, as there are systems of production where lower growth rates can be accepted and yet profitability maintained.

Under British conditions, lamb feeding systems designed to maximize lamb growth rate fall into two categories: early weaning on to cereal diets, or finishing from quality grazing and the ewe's milk. The early weaning of lambs on to a cereal diet depends on encouraging early development of the rumen, and the introduction of the lamb to solid food at an early age will encourage this development. Some growth check is to be expected when the lambs are weaned, but subsequently high growth rates and food conversion efficiencies can be expected.

Achieving maximal growth rates at grass depends on the provision of high quality pasture and a good supply of ewe's milk. Generally speaking this is difficult to achieve with twins or in the harsher areas of Britain. Nevertheless, this system is practised by some extremely efficient producers in lowland Britain.

Lamb feeding systems designed to achieve less than maximal rates of gain incorporate some method of limiting energy and/or protein intake. This may be due to natural factors, such as the quality of available grazings or the level of the ewe's milk yield in relation to the lamb's requirements, or artificially created as part of the system by heavier stocking. Whatever the method used, it is essential to maintain certain minimal levels of nutrient intake in order to achieve some growth. The level of energy intake will determine growth rate but the quality of the food being eaten will affect appetite levels. Thus energy requirements cannot be separated from factors which influence intake. The requirements for protein are also important. Below about 100 g/kg DM of crude protein in the diet the rumen microflora will not be able to function properly. Although in some circumstances the actual requirements of the lamb may be less than this in terms of the protein necessary for tissue growth, intake must not fall below this level if growth is to occur.

Lamb survival

The survival of the new born lamb is largely dependent on good birthweight and a vigorous maternal response from the ewe. The heavy demands on the ewe prior to parturition and in early lactation have been referred to in connection with optimum ewe nutrition, and the importance of efficient feeding during this period must be stressed. Despite all efforts there will be a proportion of unthrifty lambs at birth in all but the very best managed flocks. Indeed, on a national level there is plenty of evidence to suggest that lamb losses are high. Recent surveys of different cases of lamb death suggest that British producers lose every fifth lamb born shortly after birth. Of the total losses it has been estimated that 40% are due to abortion in late pregnancy and still-births and 30% to exposure and starvation.

This latter group, probably somewhere in excess of one million lambs per year, represent significant increases in flock output if they can be saved. An understanding of the condition of hypothermia, the principle reason for such deaths, can help producers plan a life saving campaign. Hypothermia means a below normal body temperature. Once the lamb's body temperature drops one or two degrees below the normal body temperature it is at risk, and unless remedial action is taken the drop continues and the lamb dies.

Certain groups of lambs are more susceptible to hypothermia than others: those from ewes in poor condition, from very young or old ewes, from large litters, from difficult births and those born under extreme climatic conditions. Two critical periods are recognisable. The first is the period from birth to five hours of age when the wet lamb loses body heat rapidly, and the second from twelve hours to three days of age when body heat is lost through starvation. Treatment depends on the age of the lamb and its body temperature. Young lambs at a temperature between 37°C and 39°C should be fed with a stomach tube and given shelter, while young lambs up to five hours old and with a temperature below 37°C should be dried and placed in a lamb warming box. Older lambs with temperatures below 37°C require an intra-peritoneal injection of glucose and then warming in a lamb warming box.

Provided that producers are aware of these requirements and are ably equipped, many of the lambs at risk can be saved.

Ewe replacements

In all sheep production systems a proportion of lambs are retained for use as parents of the next generation. If ewe replacements are to be mated as ewe lambs they require a high nutritional level in order to attain puberty at seven to eight months of age. At mating they should be at least 60% of their expected mature liveweight. Higher weights are generally associated with earlier puberty, a stronger oestrus cycle and better ovulation.

Lamb marketing

In general, market requirements for lamb carcases can be described in terms of carcase weight, fatness and conformation. In many countries simple descriptive systems of carcase characteristics are available. These can be used by producers to meet the requirements of their own particular markets more precisely and by meat traders as a common language of trade from the producer through to the retail end of the marketing chain. The success of these carcase description or classification schemes is mixed. In France, for example, all lambs are classified and a number of producer owned abattoirs make incentive payments to producers on the basis of the classification, but the enthusiasm for the scheme amongst meat wholesalers is minimal.

Carcase description
Carcase description in Britain is operated by MLC on an optional basis. Currently some 33% of the national lamb kill is classified but because the scheme is adopted by only some abattoir owners the availability of the scheme to individual producers varies around the country. The scheme is, however, widely quoted in the industry and its principles are generally understood by producers.

Classification is a description of fat content and carcase shape which, when combined with weight, gives a valid description of the carcase which can provide an acceptable medium of communication between producers and wholesalers. Fatness is defined on a scale of 1 to 5 ranging from very lean to very fat, classes 3 and 4 are divided into low (L) and high (H). Visual appraisal of the external fat cover (subcutaneous fat) is used to determine fat class. The range of subcutaneous fat levels and amount of total fat in the carcase are given in Table 4.13.

Shape, or conformation, is divided into five classes (EUROP) ranging from E for extra conformation, through average (R) and poor (O), to very poor (P). Conformation class is estimated by visual appraisal, taking into account carcase blockiness and fullness of the

Table 4.13 Fatness in the MLC classification scheme. (Source: MLC)

MLC fat class	% of total carcase weight	
	Subcutaneous fat	Total fat
1	under 6	14.3
2	6.0–9.9	20.5
3	10.0–13.9	26.6
4	14.0–17.9	32.7
5	over 17.9	38.9

legs. Typical carcase shapes for each conformation class are shown in Fig. 4.6.

The resulting grid of fatness by conformation gives a total of twenty-nine classification categories. A lamb at fat class 3L and in the E conformation category for example, would be described as 3LE. The percentage of classified carcases falling into each category in 1992 is shown in Fig. 4.7.

Once a system such as the sheep carcase classification scheme described above has been developed, it can have benefits throughout

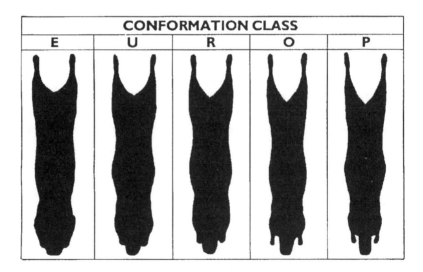

Fig. 4.6 Conformation classes in the MLC classification scheme. (Source: MLC, 1989)

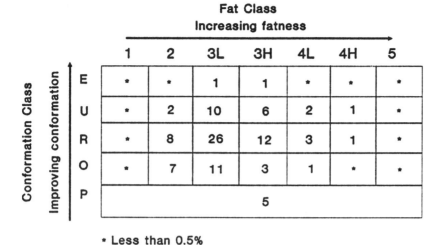

Fig. 4.7 MLC sheep carcase classification grid (the percentage of classified carcases falling into each category in 1992). (Source: Cuthbertson, 1993)

the marketing chain. The requirements of meat traders can be easily defined for producers, who in turn can gauge the type of carcase they are producing. The buying and selling grades used by wholesalers can be defined and used to check correct procurement and distribution to retail outlets. Classification can also aid retailers to describe their requirements, compare wholesalers' quotations and improve returns by reducing trimming losses and checking the specification of delivered carcases. At the time of writing a mandatory EC classification scheme has been announced to apply in member states from April 1993. Whilst firm details had yet to be agreed it was likely that the new scheme would not differ significantly from the existing MLC one. The development of sheep carcase classification is not an end in itself, of course, and producers must be able to grow lambs to meet the requirements of the meat trade.

Market requirements
In Britain market requirements vary according to regional preferences, but overall needs can be identified. A wide band of carcase weights are acceptable, from 16 kg to 20 kg with lighter and heavier lambs also being accepted on certain markets. British producers must, in addition, consider export markets. Weight preferences in some of the more important markets for British lamb are given in Table 4.14.

Table 4.14 General market requirements for British lamb. (Source: MLC)

Carcase weight (kg)	Market proportion (%)	Market outlet
Under 12	5	Italy, Spain
12–16	25	Britain, Spain, Greece
16–20	50	Britain, France, Belgium, Switzerland
Over 20	20	Britain, Belgium, Switzerland, Germany

Carcase fatness requirements are for fat classes 2 and 3L. Fatness has given some reason for concern in recent years in Britain and, with positive indications that consumers object to excessive amounts of fat, considerable efforts have been made to reduce levels of carcase fatness.

The importance of producing carcases of low levels of fatness is emphasized when the saleable meat yield is considered. In Table 4.15 figures are presented for each fat class of the MLC scheme. Between fat classes 2 and 4 there is a difference of 3½% in the proportion of saleable meat in the carcase. In addition, there is 6% less lean meat in the saleable meat of the fatter carcase. The amount of fat trimmed from carcases varies between retailers depending on their trades, but clearly the amount of trim is greater for carcases at the fatter end of the scale.

The difference is significant for the consumer, too. For example, a 1 kg half shoulder of lamb from a fat class 4 carcase that has already been trimmed contains an extra 100 gm of fat. This will probably be left on the side of the dinner plate.

The lamb cutting methods discussed in Chapter 2 produce a range of boneless cuts which allow more fat trimming than does conventional lamb butchery. When prepared as boneless cuts, fat class 2 or 3L lambs have a saleable meat yield of around 70% (fat trim of 9%) compared with 64.5% (fat trim of 16%) for fat class 4 lambs. Despite the extra fat trimming which the boneless technique permits, there is still considerable inter-muscular fat which cannot be removed without the risk of cutting into the muscles or through the skin. Thus even after extra trimming the boneless cuts and joints from fat class 4L carcases are fatter than those from fat classes 2 or 3L carcases, and they look much less attractive. New methods of presentation are an essential element in improving the demand for lamb among younger

Table 4.15 Yield of saleable meat according to fat class. (Source: MLC, 1989)

	MLC Fat class						
	1	2	3L	3H	4L	4H	5
	(percentage of carcase weight)						
Saleable meat	95	93	92	91	90	89	85.5
Fat trim	4	6	7	8	9	10	13.5
Other trim	1	1	1	1	1	1	1
	(percentage of saleable meat)						
Lean	67.5	64	62	60	59	57	56
Fat	10.5	16	18.5	21	24	26	29
Bone	22	20	19.5	19	18	16	15

consumers but they can only be effectively applied to lambs in fat classes 2 or 3L. Since 1977 the proportion of classified carcases falling into classes 4 and 5 has fallen from 14% to 7%, indicating the willingness of producers to respond to market demands.

Conformation requirements are a little less precise than those for fatness and weight, being confounded to some extent with fatness. It is held by some people that the shape of the carcase gives an idea of the lean meat content with thicker, blockier carcases having more lean meat than poorly shaped carcases. Conformation as a predictor of lean percentage in the carcase has, however, been studied and found to be of little value (Kempster, Croston & Jones, 1982). Nevertheless there is no doubt that the meat trade places a higher value on a carcase of good shape, presumably because it is more pleasing to the eye. General market requirements are therefore for extra conformation.

Specifications
Producers can only produce to the requirements of the market if their customers, the abattoirs and meat wholesalers, provide a specification to which some reasonable financial incentives are attached. Nationally there are some problems because 70% of finished lambs are sold through live auction markets where it is difficult to operate any kind of specification system. Nevertheless, there are now a number of major abattoirs offering some kind of detailed specification. An

Table 4.16 Carcase prices by conformation and fat class. Prices (p/kg carcase weight) for lamb carcases of 15–18.4 kg from a sample of abattoirs in a sample period, January 1993. (Source: Cutherbertson, 1993)

	Fat class						
Conformation	1	2	3L	3H	4L	4H	5
E	—	+10	+10	—	—	—	—
U	—	+3	+3	–4	—	—	—
R	—	+3	—	–7	–27	—	—
O	—	–6	–1	–12	–40	—	—
P	—	—	—	—	—	—	—

example price schedule based on the MLC classification grid is given in Table 4.16. These prices are paid on a weight range of 15–18.4 kg deadweight and the prices given refer to the amount per kg.

Actual specifications will depend upon the requirements of individual buyers, which will vary. Their existence is, however, a positive force in lamb marketing and many producers are able to utilize them to their own financial advantage.

Selecting lambs for slaughter
Once they are aware of the requirements and any particular specifications which may be of value, producers can plan to meet their markets. Two main factors can help them produce lambs which fall into the market target area: the selection of sires with good performance and good conformation from a suitable terminal ram breed, and the selection of lambs for slaughter at the correct level of finish. The producer must therefore estimate accurately the lamb's weight and carefully assess its level of fatness.

Lamb weight
The breed liveweight is not a precise guide for individual lambs but it is a reliable guide to the average fatness of batches of lambs within a breed type. Lambs that have grown well, without a check, will normally produce carcases in fat class 3 in MLC's Sheep Carcase Classification Scheme and will kill-out at about 48% when slaughtered at half their potential adult breed liveweight. As a general guide, lambs slaughtered about 10% above or below the predicted slaughter weight of a particular breed or cross will classify 4 or 2 for fatness

respectively. For example, Suffolk × Mule lambs slaughtered at 43 kg liveweight tend to produce 20.5 kg carcases of MLC fat class 3. Slaughtered at 47 kg or 40 kg, similar lambs would produce carcase weights of 22.5 kg and 19 kg and would classify 4 and 2 respectively for fatness.

A further factor is the sex of the lamb. Ewe lambs are fatter than wether lambs of the same breed at the same weight. To achieve the same level of fatness wether lambs should be killed at 5% above the average slaughter weight and ewe lambs at 10% below the average. Hoggets have lower lifetime weekly gains than lambs and so can generally be taken to slightly heavier weights and remain in the same fat class; the difference is about 5%.

The breed liveweight is the average of mature ram and ewe weights. Information on adult liveweights of breeds can be used to indicate the liveweight of lambs required to produce carcases in the target range. This applies to any particular breed or combination of breeds. Breed liveweights for the numerically important breeds are shown in Table 4.17. The potential adult liveweight of a lamb lies mid-way between the breed weights of its parents.

Table 4.17 Breed liveweights. (Source: MLC, 1989)

Terminal sire breeds	kg	Shortwools	kg
Dorset Down	77	Devon Closewool	66
Hampshire Down	78	Dorset Horn	82
Île de France	78	Clun Forest	73
Oxford Down	100		
Southdown	61		
Suffolk	91	*Hillbreeds*	
Texel	87		
Charollais	86	Cheviot	64
		North Country Cheviot	82
		Scottish Blackface	70
Longwools		Swaledale	64
		Welsh Mountain	50
Bluefaced Leicester	96		
Border Leicester	94		
Devon and Cornwall Longwool	95		
Lincoln Longwool	91		
Romney Marsh	77		
Teeswater	96		

NB   Breed liveweights of crossbreds are the averages of the parent breed liveweights.

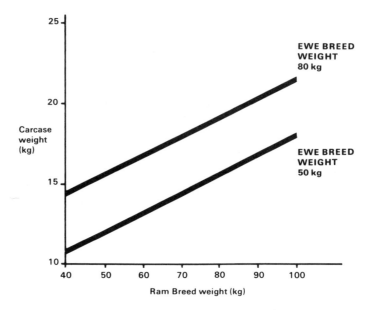

Fig. 4.8 General relationship between breed weights and carcase weights at fat class 3. (Source: MLC, 1989)

A given carcase weight can be produced from a number of ewe/ram breed combinations (Fig. 4.8) and the final choice of breeds must depend upon the suitability of the cross to fit into an overall production strategy.

Fatness assessment
While potential adult weights are a valuable guide to predicting slaughter weights, success ultimately depends upon skill in selecting individual lambs on the farm. Practice in handling live lambs to assess individual fatness levels is therefore essential and, until the experience is acquired, carcases from each batch sent for slaughter should be examined at the abattoir. If a visit to the abattoir is not possible then carcase classification results can be used to show how accurate the selection for fatness has been. Four points on a lamb will provide a reliable guide to the fatness of its carcase when handled (Fig. 4.9). The two most important areas are around the tail root or dock (A) and along the spinous processes of the back bone over the eye muscle and tips of the transverse processes in the lumbar region (B). Handling over the spinous processes of the back bone over the shoulder (C) and along the breast bone (D) are only used as an additional guide.

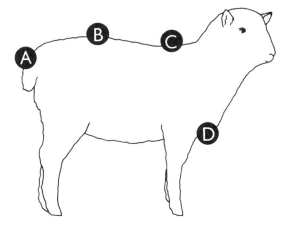

Fig. 4.9 Lamb handling points. (Source: MLC, 1989)

A diagram of the cut surface of the loin at the third/fourth vertebrae is presented in Fig. 4.10 to illustrate the fat cover over the eye muscle in carcases of fat classes 2 and 4. Based on the handling characteristics at A and B, an overall score for fatness from 1 (leanest) to 5 (fattest) can be made similar to the fat scale of the MLC classification scheme. The handling characteristics for each fat class at the loin and dock are presented in Table 4.18.

The handling technique can be used to assess the fatness of all breeds, but it is important to allow for differences in thickness of wool.

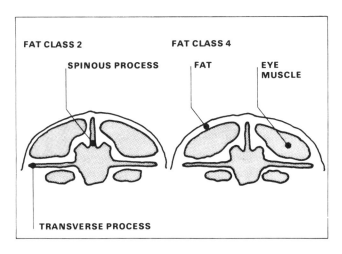

Fig. 4.10 Cross section through lumbar region of lambs at two fat levels. (Source: MLC, 1989)

Table 4.18 Lamb handling characteristics at different fat classes. (Source: MLC, 1989)

Fat class	Dock	Loin
1	Fat cover very thin. Individual bones very easy to detect.	Spinous processes very prominent. Individual processes felt very easily. Transverse processes prominent. Very easy to feel between each process.
2	Fat cover thin. Individual bones detected easily with light pressure.	Spinous processes prominent. Each process is felt easily. Transverse processes – each process felt easily.
3	Individual bones detected with light pressure.	Spinous and transverse processes – tips rounded. With light pressure individual bones felt as corrugations.
4	Fat cover quite thick. Individual bones detected only with firm pressure.	Spinous processes – tips of individual bones felt as corrugations with moderate pressure. Transverse processes – tips detected only with firm pressure.
5	Fat cover thick. Individual bones cannot be detected even with firm pressure.	Spinous and transverse processes – individual bones cannot be detected even with firm pressure.

It is also important to apply minimum pressure with the fingers to avoid bruising which can seriously lower the financial value of carcases.

Carcase damage
Selection of lambs to meet the requirements of the market cannot be undertaken successfully without careful handling. A feature of any practical training exercise which involves handling live lambs in a lairage and subsequently inspecting the carcases are the comments from producers about carcase damage. Most producers in Britain never see the carcases they produce and therefore are unaware of the

level of damage arising through either bad handling or careless injection techniques.

Bruising and vaccination abscesses devalue the carcase, particularly if they occur in the high price areas. These blemishes have to be cut away, reducing carcase value considerably. Producers can minimize these problems through careful lamb handling and correct vaccination.

Vaccination should be carried out as hygienically as possible and always in the upper third of the neck (scrag), thus avoiding the high price cuts (Fig. 4.11). Frequent changes of needle are necessary – after every twenty-five sheep and always when there has been a break in the work. Sheep should be clean and dry, otherwise the needle very quickly becomes contaminated.

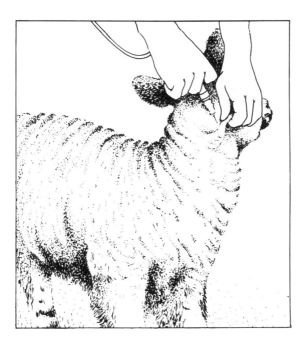

Fig. 4.11 Vaccination site to avoid carcase damage. (Source: MLC, 1984)

The genetic improvement of animal resources

Management improvements to increase output often require the provision of extra resources, and these need to be maintained if the extra output is not to be lost. Genetic improvements, on the other hand, provide the possibility of increased output from existing resources. Once a genotype has been improved the benefits remain within the system at no further cost.

The basis of genetic improvement is exploitation of the genetic variation which occurs naturally in all quantitative traits. Improvements in performance can be made by accurately identifying the genetically superior animals in a population for a particular trait or combination of traits and then using them as parents of the next generation. A considerable body of genetic theory and animal breeding practice has been founded on this simple concept, and can be divided into two broad categories: methods attempting to identify superior genotypes and methods attempting to utilize the superior genotypes thus identified in the most efficient manner. Successful improvement programmes consist of three essential elements: clear definition of the selected objectives, accurate methods of identifying superior genotypes, and practical schemes which allow the superior genetic material to be used advantageously.

Selection objectives

The problem with most breeding schemes is the endless list of objectives which individual breeders have. Careful definition of objectives which are achievable and relevant to the future of the particular breed is critically important. A number of general points can be made but ultimately it is the individual breeder, faced with his own circumstances, who must make the final choice.

Performance records, either singly or gathered together into appropriate selection indices, should be the sole basis for selection. However, the sheep produced has to be presented to potential buyers as attractively as possible if a sale is to be achieved. Many breeders tend to over emphasize this point and place too much importance on the appearance of sheep at a show or sale. If the selection objectives are chosen for reasons of increased or more efficient production, the look of the animal is a worthless guide to superiority and should in fact be played down. Regretfully, very few breeders in Britain and probably in many other countries can afford to neglect the appearance of their sheep and select solely on performance since their markets force them to attend to 'breed type'. That being the case, breeders must acknowledge this as a weakness of their selection programme and accept that they may be losing a little in the efficient selection of animals for production characteristics.

Breeders participating in MLC's improvement programmes are

asked to assess their own objectives regularly. For example, one group of Welsh Mountain breeders involved in a group breeding scheme (CAMDA) put together a set of objectives for their nucleus breeding flock following many months of careful analysis and individual assessment. Their final objectives are now clearly understood by all, and this has enabled their advisors to put together a successful yet practical breed improvement plan. These objectives are presented in Table 4.19 with an indication of the relative amount of progress achieved for each when selection is based on a five character index. The maximum progress which could be achieved for a single objective is 1.0. An analysis of their selection response on 12 week weight after several years demonstrated an annual genetic gain of 0.42 kg per annum (Guy, Croston, Jones, Williams & Cameron, 1986).

Identifying superior genotypes
Techniques such as performance testing, progeny testing, the use of contemporary comparisons, Best Linear Unbiased Prediction (BLUP) and selection indices are all concerned with trying to estimate the true breeding value of individual animals. Each technique has a place in livestock improvement programmes, depending on a range of different factors both biological and economic. Techniques which are of great value in one farm species may be totally irrelevant in another.

Performance testing
Performance testing is an adequate method of estimating the breeding value of an individual when the genotype of the animal is well correlated with its phenotype. Such characters of moderate to high heritability include fleece weight, body weight and early lamb growth rate in sheep. The aim of the test is to reduce the environmental effects on the tested animals to a minimum, both on the test and in the pre-test environment. Thus the conditions for expressing the trait under consideration are made as similar as possible for all animals.

Table 4.19 Relative progress for each of four selection objectives in the CAMDA scheme

Growth	0.54
Maternal growth	0.20
Mature size	0.38
Litter size	0.02

Performance testing is a feature of many national sheep improvements schemes but does not feature regularly in British programmes. Central performance tests for growth rate, feed conversion efficiency and conformation are found, in particular, in Germany where they provide means of assessing breeding values which would not be possible in individual flocks because of small flock size. In Britain many terminal sire breed flocks are big enough to provide large groups of contemporaries for comparative purposes and the extra cost of central facilities cannot be justified. MLC has co-operated in a number of central performance tests involving early weaning of ram lambs at two to three days of age and artificially rearing them on milk replacer up to thirty days. Lambs are subsequently tested on high energy complete diets for a period of 100–120 days. This type of test has been shown to be practical and to increase the accuracy of breeding values. However, little interest in the technique was forthcoming from breeders. In the mid-1980s a group at the East of Scotland College, Edinburgh (now part of the Scottish Agricultural College) started a Suffolk selection flock to study the relationship between body composition and other performance traits under intense selection for lean tissue growth rate. They opted for an intensive performance test routine to maximize their progress (Simm, Dingwall, Murphy & Brown, 1990).

Progeny testing
When the genetic influence on a trait is not well expressed in the individual, when carcase traits are of interest or when a character is sex-linked, progeny testing can be employed to give an estimate of an individual's breeding value. As the name implies, it is the offspring of the test animal that are measured and the results related back to the sire. Progeny testing is used widely in improvement programmes and two notable examples merit some discussion.

In Norway, ram circles are organized to progeny test teams of ram lambs which have been selected for testing on their own performance. The characters of interest relate to growth and carcase characteristics and currently over 2000 rams are progeny tested annually. Reliable estimates of annual rates of progress have been calculated and the efficiency of this system under Norwegian conditions is undisputed. The general aspects of the Norwegian ram circles will be discussed further, later in this chapter.

Two breed societies in France, Île de France and Texel, have adopted progeny testing as their means of assessing ram breeding values. The overall Île de France programme is too complex to discuss in detail here. Where progeny testing is concerned, however, rams are tested independently in one of two ways. Daughters produced by AI in breeders' flocks are monitored for three lambings and the rams are then assessed on their daughters' litter size and milking ability. At the same time, again through AI, the rams are progeny tested in a central flock of Berrichon du Cher × Romanov ewes and the growth and carcase characteristics of the resulting lamb crop evaluated.

However valuable any progeny test is in a programme, there are two main disadvantages; the first being the elapsed time between the start of the test and results becoming available, and the second being the cost of the testing facilities. These two factors account for the lack of real involvement in progeny testing in Britain. In the late 1970s MLC was actively involved with the British Texel Society in progeny testing a team of ten to twelve rams each year, but the cost and time involved became prohibitive and all efforts have now ceased. This quite naturally places restrictions on the objectives which can be considered by breeders. Although terminal sire breeders must, by virtue of the role played by their rams in the British lowland sheep industry, take an interest in monitoring carcase characteristics, the reality of the situation is that unless they are prepared to progeny test they have little chance of improvement in these characters.

Best linear unbiased prediction
Recent developments in computer technology have made the use of advanced statistical techniques a more practical alternative to progeny or performance testing. Best linear unbiased prediction (BLUP) methods can be used to predict the breeding value of any group of animals that are genetically linked and have been recorded for any traits of interest. BLUP has been used extensively in dairy industries where the use of AI sires is common and thus many herds are genetically linked. In many sheep industries such linking is uncommon. However, recent developments in the use of sire referencing schemes have enabled a much wider comparison of animals to be made, in fact, between all recorded animals and their ancestors in all linked flocks. BLUP can also be used in ram circles and group breeding schemes (see later) to compare all recorded animals (Croston & Guy, 1990).

Carcase assessment on the live animal
It is impossible to measure potential carcase composition on the live animal. All techniques employed to estimate carcase composition of

the live animal rely on the relationships between live animal measurements and some measures of carcase composition. In practice, the accuracy of these relationships is set against the cost of obtaining the live animal measurements. Allen (1990) reviewed a wide range of techniques available to predict carcase composition in lambs. Only a few of them have been used on enough live animals to obtain useful relationships between live and carcase measurements (see for example Simm, 1987). Only three methods have ever proved cost effective to use in sheep breeding programmes, the weigh scale, the A-mode scanner and the ultrasonic scanner. In 1988, following the pioneering work of Simm and colleagues, MLC introduced an ultrasonic scanning service (Croston & Owen, 1992).

In a MLC trial which employed a wide range of visual assessments, linear body measurements and ultrasonic scans to assess body composition in six month old Suffolk rams, none of these improved the prediction of carcase lean content and lean gain per day over and above the easily obtained data of liveweight and age (Cuthbertson, Croston & Jones, 1983).

Simm (1987) describes a comparative trial, including a range of ultrasound machines and X-ray computed tomography, to take live animal measurements on a group of animals which were later slaughtered and their actual carcase composition assessed. Ultrasound measurements of fat and muscle depth increased the accuracy of predicting lean content of the carcase by 16% over using liveweight alone. X-ray computed tomography was 32% more accurate. Whilst the tomograph has potential to more accurately identify animals of good carcase composition it is an expensive technique to operate and it is more common to find ultrasound machines being used to estimate carcase composition.

On farm evaluation of genetic merit
Accurately identifying genetically superior animals is not easy because the genotype of the animal is influenced to varying degrees by the environment. Measurements can only be made on the overall appearance of the animal, its phenotype. The heritability of a character is the measurement of the variation which can be attributed to the animal's complement of genes and which is, therefore, passed on to the next generation. Estimates of heritability for the more important traits in British flocks are presented in Table 4.20.

Environmental influences are particularly important in the prediction of breeding values. For example, eight week lamb weights are

Table 4.20 Heritability estimates for important traits

	Heritability (%)
Mature size	15–55
Litter size	10–20
Milk yield	10–20
Growth rate	10–30
Weight at eight weeks	14–20
Carcase composition	25–50
Conformation	25–50
Fleece weight	30–40
Fleece quality	40–70

influenced by age of ewe, sex of lamb, birth rearing type and date of birth. These factors can account for over 45% of observed variation in eight week lamb weights. If the variation can be removed by statistical means, therefore, the possibility of measuring the genotype of individual animals more accurately is increased.

Selection criteria, the characters actually measured, are influenced by environmental effects such as age of ewe or sex of lamb. Failure to take account of these environmental factors where they are known to influence the character under consideration will lead to lower rates of genetic gain because the breeding values produced will be less accurate. This is particularly important where characters of ewe reproduction or lamb growth are involved. Any improvement programme therefore requires some type of recording scheme so that necessary performance data can be collected on an individual animal basis and adjusted for these environmental effects. A number of schemes are operated in Europe and these have been reviewed by Croston *et al.* (1980). In New Zealand and Australia similar official recording schemes are available to producers, but wool records play an important part in those schemes compared to schemes operated in Europe.

The MLC Sheepbreeder scheme is a general scheme which can be used for any of the breeds found in Britain (MLC, 1992a). In addition to ewe mating and lambing details, the weights of lambs are recorded at various stages through the year. In terminal sire breed flocks lambs are weighed and scanned at twenty-one weeks of age. In the remaining flocks lambs are weighed at eight to ten weeks of age, or at ten to twelve weeks for hill flocks. Environmental effects are eliminated through the use of standardized contemporary comparisons. For a given character, animals are only compared with those animals experiencing the same environmental effects. When considering early lamb growth, for example, a twin born ram lamb out of an old ewe is compared to the average of all twin born ram lambs out of ewes and his superiority or inferiority is expressed in standard deviation units above or below the common environmental group mean. This value is then used as a criterion in the selection indices which are produced.

Both performance and progeny testing attempt to reduce environmental effects on the traits of interest by influencing the physical environment of the measured animals. The use of both contemporary comparisons and BLUP are alternative means of reducing environmental differences by statistical means. Specific environmental effects are estimated using complex mathematical procedures and the estimated breeding values of an individual arrived at by adjusting the value of the recorded trait according to the estimated environmental effects.

When more than one trait is of importance in a selection programme it is possible to define the genotype that is to be improved in terms of a selection index which combines all the required traits. The selection objective is thus to improve the composite breeding value of the traits in the index, which are often weighted by some economic measure. The selection criteria may be all or some of the traits in the composite genotype. The breeding value of the selection objective is estimated from the selection criteria using previously determined genetic and economic relationships.

Two types of selection index are produced by MLC: a single character index based on eight week lamb weight and used to estimate breeding values of ewe and ram lambs, and a more complex selection index involving several characters which will be used to estimate the lamb's breeding value for a variable combination of objectives. The evaluation of breeding stock within the MLC Sheepbreeder scheme is summarized in Table 4.21.

Breeding values produced in schemes such as this are only strictly comparable within the flock of origin or genetically linked flocks.

Utilizing superior animals in breeding programmes

Two important factors influence the rate of progress which can be made in an improvement programme: the selection intensity and the generation interval.

The selection intensity is the proportion of the replacements

Table 4.21 Evaluation of breeding stock within MLC's Sheepbreeder scheme.

Breed type	Improvement objectives	Estimated breeding value		
		Estimator	Animal type	Source of information
Multi-purpose of ewe breeds (e.g. Lleyn)	Growth rate Prolificacy Milking ability Mature size	Ewe index – Multi-character index	Lamb	Individual, half-sibs, parents and grandparents
Terminal sire (e.g. Suffolk)	Growth rate	Lamb weight – Eight-week weight combined in a single character index	Lamb	Individual and half-sibs
	Lean growth	Lean index – Fat and muscle depths plus liveweight	Lambs at 6 months age	Individual and half-sibs

retained out of all available candidates, e.g. one ram lamb out of every twelve born or one ewe lamb out of every four born. The group size from which one replacement is selected has a direct bearing on the relative genetic progress which can be achieved (Fig. 4.12). Most attention is paid to this on the ram side, but significant improvements

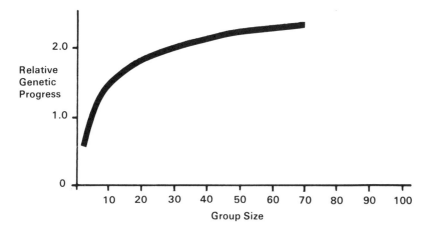

Fig. 4.12 Effect of group size on genetic progress when selecting the same number of replacements

in progress can be made if the selection intensity is increased on the ewe side. For example, if the selection intensity is increased from one ewe replacement out of five to one out of ten then the response in progress is almost double.

Generation interval, i.e. the average age of the parents when replacement lambs are born, determines the speed at which the genetic material in the population is changed. The shorter the generation interval, the greater the annual rate of progress. In a typical flock replacing rams annually, ram age is one year and ewe age is around three and a half to four and a half years, giving a generation interval of 2.4 years.

Breeders often ask what rates of progress they can expect or, after a number of years of selection, what progress has been achieved. There are two methods available to breeders which allow progress to be assessed, both rely on certain specialized techniques. The use of a genetically unselected control flock, run with the main breeding flock, can be used to monitor improvements in the selected flock. This is an expensive method but has been used successfully in some situations. It is also possible to use BLUP to estimate the breeding value of animals and compare the trends in breeding values of all new lambs every year. A number of good examples from selection experiments show where genetic progress has been measured. Those dealing with selection for an increase in the numbers of lambs born show a marked and uniform rate of response at about 1.5% per annum (Land, Atkins & Roberts 1983). Despite the low heritability of this character, the large variation in litter size enables reasonably significant gains to be made in the long term. Simm (1992) has reviewed responses to selection in weight-for-age and ultrasound measurements of fat and muscle depth and found responses ranging from 0.4 to 4.5% per year.

The time and effort spent on detailed recording is only of value if the superior breeding animals are utilized effectively, and this implies the need for a comprehensive breeding plan which will maximize genetic progress. Many breeders participating in recording schemes are unable to make this final commitment or use their information to initiate flock improvement schemes.

Flock size is always a limiting feature. In the MLC scheme average flock size is currently 120 ewes, ranging from 20 ewes to over 600 ewes. Small flocks are not all necessarily participating for genetic reasons. Some record for the simple reason of involvement. However, smaller flocks with aspirations to select within their own flock are hampered by a lack of contemporaries in the various environment categories.

Consequently their within flock comparisons are unreliable. In larger flocks, on the other hand, the maintenance of records may be counterproductive. In large extensive hill flocks there is little possibility of detailed individual ewe records being collected and prospects for within flock selection are therefore limited. Before discussing practical systems of overcoming these problems of extremes in flock size, however, normal within flock selection schemes can be considered.

Inbreeding can be a problem, particularly in small flocks, when a within flock policy is followed and to minimize the problem a simple family breeding system is advocated. Initially the flock is divided into five or six equal groups of ewes (genetically equal if possible, and numerically equal). Replacements are selected within family, the ewe lambs remaining in the family of their mother while the best ram lambs are moved into the next family (Fig. 4.13). This procedure is repeated annually and, provided a ram is only used for two years and only one ram is taken from a ewe, inbreeding is minimized for several generations.

The merits of this system are that it is easy to operate on the ground and that it forces breeders to look at their selection decisions in a systematic and planned way. There is no need for the flock to remain closed provided that any rams introduced from outside are selected on

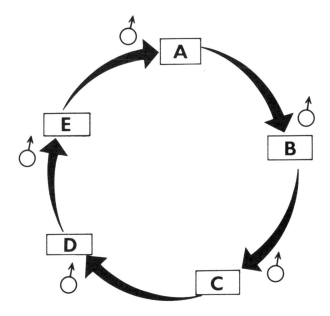

Fig. 4.13 Family breeding programme. (Source: MLC)

the same sound principles of performance. If they are superior to the home bred stock their progeny will subsequently be selected in the system on their own merits.

Within flock selection

Flocks ranging from 150 ewes to 600 ewes are able to operate useful selection programmes of their own. Breeders' reports produced in the MLC scheme are designed to assist breeders in these selection decisions and MLC advisors are on call to discuss aspects of selection policy.

Selection objectives for terminal sire breeders are improved carcase quality, i.e. more lean at a given age. The MLC Lean Index, based on weight, ultrasound fat depth and muscle depth at the 3rd lumbar vertebra, is a useful estimate of lean and fat content of the animal at 21 weeks of age. Selection objectives for ewe breed or dual purpose breeds will vary according to the specific requirements of breeders but include mature size, prolificacy, milking ability and lamb growth rate. Genetic progress is achieved by selecting ewe and ram replacements from the highest rated animals and, if flock circumstances allow, by culling ewes which have the lowest genetic merit. Higher rates of progress are achieved if generation intervals are kept as low as possible.

Ram circles

Progeny tests involving a common set of sires over several flocks is a way of overcoming problems of small flock size which has been successfully adopted in Norway. Breeders organize themselves into ram circles and each year use a significant proportion of young rams selected from amongst their own group or from other similarly organized groups. Rams are moved from farm to farm on a daily basis with the result that progeny from each are born in all participating flocks. Flocks are fully recorded and the progeny groups evaluated on the basis of an early weight taken before the flocks are moved to the mountain pastures and on subsequent weaning weights and carcase characteristics which become available in the autumn.

Ram breeding values are available before the next mating which, for a progeny test, is very quick. The government provides financial incentives to ensure that above average rams are used in the industry, but the money is not forthcoming until a given number of ewes are mated to the ram and he has been slaughtered. This ensures a continual demand for improved stock. The elite of the progeny tested rams are reserved for planned matings to produce further sons for progeny testing.

The organization of this scheme is impressive both for its scale – over 2000 rams are progeny tested in ram circles annually – and because of its excellent organization. It has been calculated that considerable genetic progress is being achieved. Within the ram circles, lamb weaning weight is increasing at a rate of 0.247 kg per lamb annually and the number of lambs weaned per ewe is increasing at an annual rate of 0.023.

Investment in ram circles and general sheep improvement is considered cost effective. The genetic component alone is reckoned to be yielding a 31% return on capital invested.

Group breeding schemes

These schemes were first developed in New Zealand in the late 1960s by farmers trying to improve the commercial performance of their breeds. Through recording and selecting on their farms they found that it was advantageous to co-operate commercially with others in the breeding and sale of their improved stock. There are now several groups in New Zealand and Australia; one group involves over a million ewes.

Most group breeding schemes have three main features:

(1) Co-operation among breeders in running a jointly owned breeding flock (the nucleus) to produce replacement rams and possibly some females for the co-operating flocks.
(2) A two-way flow of selected rams, and possibly ewes, from the central flock to the co-operators (the base flocks) and of selected females, and possibly males, from the co-operating flocks to the central flock.
(3) Selection based on records of performance for commercially important characteristics.

The general form of a group breeding scheme is shown in Fig. 4.14. The co-operating breeders record their flocks and select the best performing females for use in the nucleus. Further recording and selection then takes place in the nucleus. The best young rams and ewes are kept for breeding in the central flock and other selected rams are used in the co-operating flocks as stock rams. While this is mainly a replacement ram breeding operation, surplus females may also be transferred. The cycle of recording and selection in both co-operating

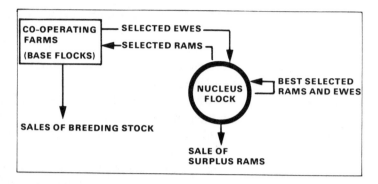

Fig. 4.14 General form of group breeding scheme. (Source: MLC, 1982a)

and central flocks continues year after year. Normally, the nucleus flock remains open to females from the co-operating flocks and is thus called an 'open nucleus'. A central flock with no females brought in from outside is known as a 'closed nucleus'.

Each group breeding scheme tends to have its own structure according to the needs and ideas of the breeders. Some schemes may be formalized and planned. Others may be rather loose agreements among breeders acting together. Some have definite rules and selection procedures, while others allow more choice for individuals.

The advantages of a group scheme can be both genetic and commercial. Where flock sizes are small there are obvious genetic advantages in increasing the scale of the breeding operation. The initial selection of sheep can create a lift in genetic merit which can be quite substantial, putting the nucleus flock above the base flocks. This genetic lift is not confined to one group as any individual could purchase genetically superior animals from individual flocks and create a high performing nucleus. The creation of the Cambridge breed is one example of such genetic screening. Ewes with exceptional litter size were brought together at Cambridge under the direction of Professor John Owen and a highly prolific breed stemmed from that original super elite group of ewes.

A major advantage of a group scheme is that it permits recording and selection effort to be concentrated in the nucleus. In hill breeds, where the extensive conditions are not conducive to individual ewe recording, this centralizing of effort can be a valuable advantage.

A number of group breeding schemes are now in operation in Britain, the most notable being the CAMDA group in North Wales. Ten Welsh Mountain breeders embarked on a group scheme in 1976 with a nucleus originally located at the ABRO Rhydeglaves farm and more latterly on a farm tenanted by the group. The central nucleus now consists of over 500 breeding ewes plus a genetic control flock which is being funded by the MAFF. Progress is encouraging, with some evidence to suggest that real genetic change is being achieved (Guy, *et al.*, 1986). The flock is MLC recorded and the group relies heavily on the breeding values produced as part of the recording scheme.

Other examples of group schemes are in North Wales with the Llyen breed, in central Wales with the Beulah Speckleface and in Kent with the Romney and Suffolk breeds. Their aims and objectives vary but all seek to gain genetic advantages through the increased scale of their operation with a nucleus flock.

Sire referencing schemes
A sire referencing scheme is one of a very limited number of methods which allow pedigree breeding animals to be genetically compared across flocks. The differences in location, climate and management experienced by physically separate flocks are enough to mask any genetic differences there may be.

Sire referencing schemes get over this problem by using a small team of common 'reference' sires by artificial insemination over all flocks. The progeny of the reference sires are related as half-sibs and have a quarter of their genes in common. These progeny are then used as a benchmark against which unrelated progeny in individual flocks can be compared. This allows all individuals in the schemes to be ranked on the same selection list, irrespective of the flock from which they come. The best out of the whole population can join the team of reference sires, while individual flocks have a choice of flock replacements from all scheme members based on good objective information. This objective information is then available to members' customers.

Sire referencing in British terminal sire flocks brings together the latest developments in artificial insemination, live animal scanning and BLUP data analysis techniques (MLC, 1991).

Schemes in the Suffolk, Charollais and Texel breeds are well established using AI for the reference sire matings. Lambs are born in December and January and are recorded in the MLC Sheepbreeder service; scanning for backfat and muscle depths takes place at 20 or 21 weeks of age in June. The scanning service provides a within-flock ranking of lambs at the time of scanning while results are collated across the scheme, aiming to provide an across-flock ranking of all animals some two weeks after the last flock's scanning visit.

Estimated breeding values
Genetic superiority for each of the measured traits is derived as Estimated Breeding Values (EBV) in the same units, taking account of:

● The three measured traits plus eight-week weights.
● All relatives and ancestors.
● Environmental differences between flocks.
● Genetic differences between flocks.

At the time of the across-flock analysis there is an immediate need to locate suitable ram lambs to join the team of reference sires in time to take semen, or to locate suitable shearling rams, before their owners sell them. A meeting of members is called to view and agree on suitable candidates and it is at this point that the group stands or falls on its ability to decide on the type of animal they are breeding towards. The most effective procedure, employed currently by the schemes, is to allow members to nominate suitable animals for group inspection over a certain standard on their record (say 160 points on the scale 0–200) and then to hold a ballot, selecting the ones upon which most members are agreed. The analysis is also able to plot the genetic change from year to year.

Reference sires are used on up to 30 ewes in each flock so it is important that a good compromise is reached between having good records and the other qualities breeders look for. The initial team of reference sires must necessarily be selected without the benefit of across-flock data, but as the schemes develop it appears that animals of good genetic merit are being located and used to good effect. The potential is there for making good genetic progress for carcase lean growth and reduced fat, making significant strides towards producing what the consumer wants.

5   Feed Resources

The digestive tract of the sheep can utilize a wide range of feeds, from milk and milk powders, cereals and high quality protein concentrates to grass, forage crops and low quality roughages. This is one of the reasons why sheep are found in such a wide range of environments. However, it is the ability to utilize the poorer quality feedstuffs which has led to the importance of sheep in world agriculture. The feeding of cereals and other high quality feeds is commonly an uneconomic proposition and in many cases leads to competition with single-stomached animals, including humans, for feed resources. In this chapter all the different types of feed will be discussed but with particular emphasis given to grazed crops, natural grassland and low quality roughages.

Grass

The most common sheep feed throughout the world is grass and grass-like species which are either grazed or fed as cut and conserved products. Grasslands used for sheep production can be classed as natural, semi-permanent or short-term, though the distinction between the three classes is not always clear.

Grazing of natural grasslands by sheep occurs in many countries. The American rangelands, the pampas of South America, large tracts of the Australian outback, the African Savannahs, Swiss Alpine pastures and the hills of Britain are just a few examples. Grazing management on these grassland areas is usually very extensive; productivity is prone to large sources of uncontrollable natural variation and the vegetation is generally self-replacing. Despite such factors, grazing management is critical in many of these areas if productivity is to be maintained. Over-grazing, for example, may lead to a deterioration in pasture quality and hence a drop in animal performance.

The term 'semi-permanent grassland' implies that while the grass-land areas may remain uncultivated for many years they were originally sown with specific species and varieties. A considerable amount of grassland in Britain falls into this category and often suffers under the misnomer 'permanent pasture'.

Short-term grassland is usually sown as part of a cropping pattern and is used, for example as a break from cereal production. The level of management of such pastures is usually the highest of the three types discussed, partly because of the more intensive nature of the farming systems in which they are found and partly due to the more accessible nature of the land utilized in this way.

Grassland in Britain

In 1992 12.6 million hectares of grassland were recorded in the UK, an area more than four times greater than the area devoted to the next most common crop, cereals. Forty-six per cent of this grassland area was rough grazing, the bulk consisting of natural vegetation; 41% was grassland over five years of age (semi-permanent pasture) and the remaining 12% was less than five years of age. This grassland was estimated to provide nearly three-quarters of the energy and protein requirements of British ruminant animals.

Distribution of grassland in Britain is very uneven. Rough grazings are more commonly found in Wales, northern England, and throughout Scotland with the exception of some eastern areas. The reverse is true of cultivated land which is predominant in the southern half of England. The grassland areas of Britain are found in Wales, south-west England, the western counties of northern England and Scotland. The distribution of grassland is closely related to several climatic factors. Potential grass yield is limited by low temperatures, drought in summer and altitude, factors which when combined can show the potential number of grass growing days available in different parts of the UK (Fig. 5.1).

The large area of eastern England shown to have less than 200 grass growing days per year suffers from both summer droughts and rela-tively cold winters. The remaining areas of Britain with less than 200 grass growing days per year are limited by the effects of altitude and winter temperatures. By contrast the western areas, with a greater number of grass growing days, are warmer and wetter areas ideally suited for grass growth. If water is not limited then a temperature of over 5.5°C is required for grass growth. Annual variation of the date in spring when temperatures rise above this level and the date in the

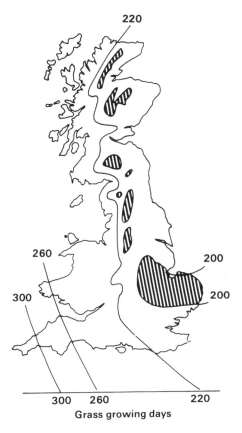

Fig. 5.1 Grass growing days in Britain. (Source: Centre for Agricultural Strategy)

autumn when temperatures fall below this level can amount to 20–30 days. The lack of water limits grass yield by about 10% for every 50 mm increase in the maximum soil water deficit.

These qualifications apart, the climatic environment of the UK is well suited to grass growing due to a consistent rainfall pattern throughout the year and a moderate range of temperatures in all seasons but winter. However, despite the suitable climatic conditions the yield of grass appears to be poor. Experimental crops under ideal conditions suggest that up to 30 tonnes of dry matter per hectare (DM/ha) could be produced. The estimated national average is above 6 t DM/ha, excluding rough grazings, and the better commercial farmers should be able to grow 20 t DM/ha.

Grass growth

Some of the factors which affect grass growth have already been mentioned but most of those that tend to be limiting are outside the control of the producer. Several other factors, however, are under the control of the grassland farmer and can be harnessed to improve grass growth. It is worth considering how grass growth manifests itself in the individual plant before considering the management factors which can affect grass growth.

The basic unit of the grass plant, the tiller, produces a continuous succession of new leaves throughout the growing season. In addition, secondary tillers are produced from the base of the primary tiller. A tiller usually contains three or four leaves and as each new leaf is formed the oldest leaf begins to die. If leaves are not harvested regularly these dead leaves represent wasted resources. Since a new leaf is produced every ten to twelve days during the grazing season, each leaf has a life of about a month. Thus if the plant is not harvested regularly a third of it is lost every ten to twelve days and the whole plant is replaced every month. At first sight the ideal situation would appear to be harvesting the grass at regular short intervals. However, grass growth is effected by the products of photosynthesis which are themselves produced in the leaf. Thus a balance must be maintained between excessive defoliation and little plant growth on the one hand and the death of leaves due to inefficient harvesting on the other.

Infrequent harvesting not only affects the quantity of leaf material collected but also leads to the growth of the stem. Stem material is usually of a lower digestibility than leaf material and the overall quality of the harvested material is thus lower under infrequent harvesting regimes. Stem elongation also increases the shading of surrounding plants, which reduces yields further and discourages secondary tiller production.

Dry matter production

The brief description of plant growth given above indicates the way in which harvesting methods can affect the yield of material removed. Frequent harvesting near to the ground will give poor yields, as will infrequent harvesting at some distance from the ground. Similarly the removal of leaves alone will produce different yields from the removal of the leaf plus stem, in terms of the quantity and quality of harvested material.

A great deal of research in grassland agronomy has been carried out using cutting as the harvesting technique. Cutting is an attractive experimental technique since defoliation can be conducted by the experimenter and the yield of cut grass easily measured. Using this technique the seasonal pattern of dry matter yield of perennial ryegrass, with unlimited water and fertilizer supply, has been shown to be bimodal, with one peak in May and a second in July. Also the quality of the grass declines through the season in terms of digestibility (D value) and crude protein content.

For obvious practical reasons few grassland agronomy trials are carried out using animals to harvest the grass. However, the pattern of dry matter production in such trials differs considerably from the bimodal pattern found in cutting work. An experiment to compare grass yields under a particular cutting regime and under continuous sheep grazing was carried out by Orr, Parsons, Treacher & Penning (1988). In this experiment maximal growing conditions were maintained by irrigation and the use of inorganic fertilizer. Three grazing treatments were applied, maintaining grass height at 3, 5 and 7 cm. Annual yields of grass organic dry-matter under grazing were 10.8, 10.1 and 8.5 t/ha for the 3, 5 and 7 cm grazed grass height treatments and 9.3 t/ha under the cutting treatment. Not only did the annual yields differ but the distribution of grass growth throughout the summer differed. The organic matter digestibility of the 3 cm sward was maintained between 82% and 86% throughout the grazing season but under less severe grazing pressure it dropped from 85% in May to 78% (5 cm) and 73% (7 cm) in August.

The results of such grazing trials have clearly demonstrated that the method of harvesting and the grazing pressure affect both the yield of grass, from any particular field, and the quality of the material harvested. Whilst cutting trials provide a reasonably straightforward method for comparing grass growth under differing growing conditions they should not be used to estimate the efficiency of utilization under grazing (Orr *et al.*, 1988).

A wealth of information about the factors which affect grass growth has been amassed over the years from cutting trials. These factors include rainfall, soil type, nitrogen and other plant nutrient usage, the variety of grass and the method of management.

Rainfall and soil type

As has already been shown, rainfall affects the number of grass growing days and hence grass yield. The higher the level of rainfall, the higher the yield. Although the response of yield to increased rainfall must eventually slow down, this rarely happens in Britain. For

Table 5.1 Grassland site classes in relation to soil type and summer rainfall. (Source: Thomas, Reeve & Fisher, 1991)

Soil texture	Average rainfall: April–September			
	More than 500 mm	425–500 mm	350–425 mm	Less than 350 mm
All soils except shallow soils over chalk/rock or gravelly and coarse sandy soils	1	2	2	3
Shallow soils over chalk or rock and gravelly and coarse sandy soils	2	3	4	5

practical purposes farms are divided into four rainfall groups in Britain: over 500 mm summer rainfall, 425–500 mm, 350–425 mm and less than 350 mm. The texture and depth of the soil also affect grass yield through water holding capacity. Farms are divided into two soil-type categories in Britain (Table 5.1). This combination of rainfall and soil type gives five site classes, each of which has particular characteristics.

Nitrogen level
The increase in grass dry matter yield with increasing nitrogen uptake appears to be linear up to about 300 kg/ha, a response of 20 kg DM per kg of additional nitrogen. Above 300 kg/ha the response to increased nitrogen use depends on the particular type of grassland under consideration. In addition, the response to nitrogen applications will depend on the level of nitrogen already in the soil. Dry matter yields for the five site classes at optimal nitrogen applications are shown in Table 5.2.

The pattern of nitrogen application affects the pattern of dry matter production throughout the season under cutting conditions. Higher applications early in the season produce a higher May peak, and higher mid-season applications give a more even dry matter production than equal applications throughout the season. In all three situations the annual yield and total nitrogen applied was the same.

Grass varieties
In Britain annual lists of recommended grass and clover varieties are published. These contain information on annual yield, persistence,

Table 5.2 Probable yields of grass when cut for conservation or to simulate grazing (based on medium N status and optimal N per cut). (Source: Thomas *et al.*, 1991)

Site class	Dry matter yield (t/ha)		
	Conserved (2 cuts at 61D)[1]	Conserved (3 cuts at 68D)[2]	Grazed
1	16.0	15.4	14.3
2	15.4	14.4	12.8
3	14.3	13.4	11.4
4	13.4	12.6	10.5
5	12.6	11.7	9.6

[1] Cuts taken on 10 June, 12 August, followed by grazing.
[2] Cuts taken on 18 May, 22 June, 27 July, followed by autumn grazing.

winter hardiness and digestibility at a suitable cutting date. The scope for increasing yields by using different varieties of grass is probably limited by the inefficient process of harvesting. Also the yields quoted for the recommended varieties are measured under cutting-only conditions and may not be a useful guide to grazing yields. The use of early grass varieties will help to spread the yield more effectively through the year and varieties which stand up to increased grazing pressure are of value.

In relation to improvements in the efficiency of sheep production that could be achieved by improved grazing management, the choice of varieties offers little scope. However, this is largely due to the vast improvements that have already been made in the plant breeding field and the resulting high yielding varieties currently available, rather than to any lack of effectiveness in the plant breeding industry.

Clover
Grass species are not the only plants used in grazed swards in Britain. Clover plays an important part too. Grazing sheep benefit directly from the presence of clover, particularly when their protein requirements are high. Lamb growth rate can be improved by the use of clover and lactating ewes can also benefit from its inclusion in the diet.

The main effect of clover on the sheep enterprise is, however, in relation to its ability to fix inorganic nitrogen from the soil. This process improves the utilization of nitrogen by the flock either by reducing the amount of nitrogen required to maintain a given level of production or by increasing the amount of herbage grown for any given level of nitrogen.

The use of grass/clover swards in Britain is widespread and the inclusion of clover in hill and upland pastures often allows the maintenance of systems of production which would otherwise not be viable. One of the important management features of such swards, however, is the problem of maintaining clover content against competition from the grass species. This is particularly crucial when conditions favour grass growth and during sward establishment. Shading by grasses represents one of the main hazards to viable clover production. The maintenance of phosphorus levels in the soil is another important factor since clovers are not able to compete well for phosphorus. Grass/clover swards require a ready supply of phosphorus in order to maintain the balance of the two species.

Excessive fertilizer nitrogen applications also adversely affect clover production, although the levels used in recorded flocks suggests that this is probably not a critical factor in sheep-grazed swards.

Interest in the use of grass/clover swards has increased in recent years due to environmental concerns with nitrogen leaching and the move to lower input agriculture. Comparative trials looking at sheep performance on grass/clover leys and all-grass leys have been carried out. Under similar conditions it appears that performance on grass/clover swards is between 75% and 100% of that on pure grass swards (Treacher, 1990). The level of performance depends on the amount of nitrogen used and on whether ewe performance is taken into account, as well as lamb growth (Vipond, Swift, McClelland & Milne, 1990).

Grass utilization
Stated simply, grassland utilization is the transfer of grass energy and protein to animal products. When planning grassland utilization, stock requirements and conservation needs must be reconciled with the expected grass growth and some allowance must be made for the annual variation in climatic conditions. Several different grazing systems, or integrated grazing and cutting systems, have been developed to improve grassland utilization. Each can be described in an idealized form but in practice many variations of each system will be found.

Grazing systems
The most common and simplest sheep grazing system in Britain is the set stocking or continuous grazing system. The sheep have access to

the same area of grass all through the grazing season. The management of the flock is straightforward once the correct levels of fertilizer application and stocking rates have been decided.

Rotational grazing systems, on the other hand, are more complicated and require a lot of management input. The grassland area is divided into a convenient number of paddocks which are then grazed and fertilized in turn. This system is more commonly used for dairy herds in Britain. The leader-follower system is a variation of the rotational grazing system where two different types of stock are to be kept on the one grass area. The stock with the higher feed requirements are let into the next paddock in advance of the second group of stock. This enables the first group to have the best of the grazing.

The 1-2-3 system integrates cutting with grazing and uses a grass area divided into three. During the early part of the season two of the divisions are closed for conservation and the third is grazed. After cutting two paddocks, one of them is then used for grazing and the other closed up for a further cut of conservation. After this cut all three are grazed until the end of the grazing season.

Buffer grazing systems have been developed to take account of the different grass yields encountered in different seasons. An area of grass (the 'buffer') is left ungrazed in the early part of the year. If conditions are such that grass is in short supply this buffer can then be used for grazing. On the other hand, if it is not required for grazing it can be cut and conserved instead. This system is tactical rather than strategic and can be included in some of the other systems if required.

Stocking rates
Some guidelines for stocking sheep during the grazing season in Britain are shown in Table 5.3. These figures combine the expected pattern of grass growth with site class, nitrogen level and the feed requirements of the flock. Additional factors such as conservation requirements and clean grazing are not included. These guidelines should be regarded as an example from which to calculate local variations. It should also be remembered that these figures are based on experimental results and that considerable variation is found in practice.

Growth and utilization interactions
So far grass growth and its utilization have been discussed in isolation, but the description given earlier clearly shows that grass growth is influenced by the method of utilization.

Table 5.3 Stocking rates during the grazing season – total weight of ewe and lamb per hectare. (Source: MLC, 1988a)

kgN/ha*	Lambing to end of July[1]	August[2]	September[3]	October[4]
	Ewe and lamb weight per ha (kg)			
Poor site				
0–75	650	1300	500	400
75–150	750	1500	600	450
150–225	900	1800	700	550
Average site				
0–75	750	1500	600	450
75–100	900	1800	700	550
150–225	1050	2100	800	650
225–300	1150	2500	950	750
Good site				
0–75	900	1800	700	550
75–150	1050	2100	800	650
150–225	1150	2500	950	750
225–300	1300	3000	1050	850

* Assumes fertilizer N applied in more or less regular amounts.
[1] Lactating ewes with lambs.   [2] Dry ewes post weaning.
[3] Preparation for mating.   [4] Mating period.

The large difference between potential grass yield and that actually harvested is partly a result of very low stocking. As stocking rate increases under continuous grazing a far greater proportion of the grass produced is harvested, but there is a fall in the amount of grass grown in the first place. The overall increase in utilization more than outweighs the decrease in the amount grown, however, and the amount harvested per hectare goes up. Grass growth may be reduced to some 18 tonnes/ha but of this some 9–10 tonnes is harvested. Note that when the sward is overstocked the rate of photosynthesis is so depressed that yield per hectare eventually falls.

Maximizing yield per hectare is unlikely to be the sole objective of the sheep producer, although getting a large proportion of the animal's diet from fresh grass is the first essential step in efficient production from grassland. Another important aim is to optimize intake and performance per head. In addition, a practical method for recognizing when intake is at its optimum is required.

Several trials have shown that the intake and performance of ewes and their twin lambs differed little in swards maintained at 6 cm, 9 cm and 12 cm although the ewes on the 6 cm sward spent a far greater proportion of the day grazing than those on the taller swards. In swards maintained at 3 cm intake was restricted; lamb growth was only marginally reduced on the 3 cm sward but the ewes lost more body condition and weight (Table 5.4).

Swards maintained at between 4 cm and 6 cm give an optimum combination of yield per head and yield per hectare, with the greatest number of animals at close to maximum intake. Looking at animal production in the spring period alone, there is little to choose between keeping the sward at 6 cm and keeping it at 9 cm or 12 cm. However, in swards kept at 9 cm and 12 cm during spring, some 50% of the tillers show stem elongation as part of the reproductive process. This increases the height at which new leaves appear in the canopy and, as grazing continues, the area of green leaf and the ability to continue to produce new leaves declines. In the experiments described above the 9 cm and 12 cm swards had no more leaf area by autumn than the one kept at 3 cm throughout but the tall swards had a large proportion of sparse, poorly rooted aerial tillers of low digestibility. Large areas of the sward were rejected and fewer animals could be sustained than on the swards kept at 3 cm or 6 cm. By contrast, in the 6 cm sward very few tillers showed appreciable stem elongation and the sward remained dense and leafy, of high digestibility and was evenly grazed (Parsons, 1984).

Table 5.4 Performance of ewes with twin lambs on swards of four heights (28 April–17 July). (Source: Penning, Parsons, Orr & Treacher, 1991)

	Sward surface height (cm)			
	3	6	9	12
Stocking rate (ewes/ha)	27.7	19.8	22.1	18.8
Intake of dry matter (kg/day)	1.67	2.65	2.59	2.71
Lamb growth rate (g/day)	210	275	260	265
Ewe liveweight loss (g/day)	188	54	42	67
Ewe loss of body condition	0.78	0.42	0.32	0.38
Time spent grazing (% of day)	53%	45%	38%	36%

By maintaining grass height at between 4 cm and 6 cm the most efficient use of grass can be made in the spring under continuous or rotational grazing systems in the spring (Grant & King, 1984). These levels of performance can be maintained if the amount of stemmy rejected grass patches are kept to a minimum by closing areas in excess of requirements for conservation. Provided the sward has been kept in good condition, it can be allowed to grow to about 8 cm in the summer to act as a buffer later in the season. Intensive grazing down to 6 cm before the pasture is rested for winter will ensure that the sward will be in good condition for the next grazing season (Maxwell & Treacher, 1987).

Grassland utilization in practice
Results from recorded flocks in Britain give a good indication of the performance obtained from grassland under commercial conditions. Such results are an amalgam of the producer's intended system, how well he achieves his objective and the effect of natural variation in a range of biological and financial factors. Consequently the range of results found in practice is large. Top third flocks, selected on the basis of gross margin per hectare, can be used to demonstrate this range (Table 5.5). Grazing season stocking rate is the most variable performance factor, with lowland flocks having a top third value 20% above the average. This is increased to 32% in upland flocks. An interesting feature of these results is that top third flocks spent more on grass production per hectare than average but on a per ewe basis they spent less than average.

The recorded levels of liveweight carried per hectare increased with

Table 5.5 Top third levels of grassland performance in lowland and upland flocks. (Source: MLC, 1984a)

	Lowland	Upland
Liveweight carried per hectare	115	123
Grazing season stocking rate	120	132
Nitrogen use per hectare	111	122
Nitrogen use per ewe	90	93
Grass cost per hectare	108	105
Grass cost per ewe	87	87

Indexed to average levels = 100.

Table 5.6 The effect of nitrogen on productivity from grass. (Source: MLC, Flockplan)

Nitrogen use (kg/ha)	Liveweight carried (kg/ha)	Gross margin per hectare*
1–50	744	100
51–100	958	111
101–150	1139	122
151–200	1251	128
201–250	1349	136
251–300	1549	146

* Indexed to 1–50 kg/ha nitrogen level = 100.

increasing nitrogen use, and this was reflected in gross margin per hectare (Table 5.6). Sheep flocks do appear to have the ability to utilize increased grass production to their advantage but the level of variation at any given nitrogen level is very high. Although differences in the productivity of short-term grassland and semi-permanent pasture can be detected in this type of data, most of the differences can be accounted for in terms of the level of nitrogen applied (Table 5.7).

The heavy dependence of sheep production on grassland in Britain means that the relationship between grassland productivity and flock profitability is very important. Increased gross margin per hectare is associated with higher stocking rates and nitrogen usage. Grassland costs per ewe, however, change very little as gross margin per hectare increases (Table 5.8).

Table 5.7 Nitrogen use and liveweight carried by pasture type. (Source: MLC, 1983)

Type of farm*	N use (kg/ha)	Liveweight carried (kg/ha)
Ley	187	1250
Permanent pasture	118	1027
No predominant type	92	905

* Farms having more than 50% of the stated pasture type.

Table 5.8 The relationship between profitability and grassland production in 1982. (Source: MLC, Flockplan)

Gross margin (£/ha)	Grazing season stocking rate (ewes/ha)	Nitrogen use (kg/ha)	Grassland cost (£/ewe)
1–100	10.5	103	4.98
101–200	11.8	128	7.26
201–300	12.3	127	6.26
301–400	14	147	5.82
401–500	15	158	5.57
501–600	16.1	159	5.32
601–700	19.1	182	5.81

Integrating conservation into a grazing system

As previously discussed, the frequent defoliation of grass at a height of 4–6 cm improves grassland utilization, provides the best quality material and maintains the sward in good condition under continuous grazing. On most grassland farms the requirements for winter feeding involve conserved grass products such as hay, silage or dried grass and these requirements must be allowed for by integrating conservation with grazing.

The timing of conservation cuts, the quality of the material removed and the grass grazing conditions all influence the efficiency of grassland utilization. Generally speaking, more frequent cutting regimes result in higher levels of grassland utilization and produce higher quality material. Although a larger interval between cuts reduces the quality of harvested material, the efficiency of grassland production increases. Separate grazing and conservation areas should be avoided since it is the successful integration of cutting and grazing which leads to improved output from grass.

Recording grassland usage

The value of physical and financial records has already been discussed in relation to the efficient operation of a flock. Similar records of grassland use and production are just as valuable and should contain as much information as possible about the grassland area on the farm (Table 5.9). Records of this type should ideally be collected for each field on the farm. However, the limitations of doing this accurately on farms may warrant a more practical grouping of grassland areas for

Table 5.9 Recorded details required to provide useful grassland records.

Grassland area.
Dates of the beginning and end of the growing season.
Type of grassland recorded, e.g. short-term, semi-permanent, grass/clover.
Variable costs of grassland production, e.g. fertilizers, seeds.
Type of stock grazing the grassland area.
Dates of grazing.
Numbers of stock grazing.
Type and quantity of conservation made from the recorded area.
Other feeds fed to the stock while at grass.

---

recording purposes. These may be conservation areas, enclosed hill, in-bye land or whatever suits a given situation.

Grassland records of this type can be used in two ways. Estimates of the cost of grazing and home-grown hay or silage can be incorporated into flock costings once they have been allocated between the enterprises utilizing the grassland. In addition, records of the physical parameters of grassland use may be used to plan future production methods and provide helpful guidelines for similar flocks elsewhere. Several different recording schemes of this type are currently in use in Britain.

The utilized metabolizable energy (UME) system estimates the metabolizable energy required by the stock grazing the recorded grassland area. Metabolizable energy fed to the stock in the form of other feeds and any conserved material removed from the grassland area and not fed to the stock is then subtracted from this amount. The remainder is assumed to be the metabolizable energy used by the grazing enterprise (see, for example, Forbes, Dibb, Green, Hopkins & Peel, 1980). This system is particularly useful in dairy enterprises where considerable amounts of concentrate feeds are fed.

Pollott & Kilkenny (1976b) described a system for recording grassland areas based on the 'livestock unit' concept. This system equates all types of grazing animals to one particular standard, the livestock unit. The livestock unit is defined as a dairy cow with certain production characteristics, in this case, and conserved products made from the recorded grassland area assume an equivalent livestock unit value. Recorded costs and areas are divided between each grazing enterprise and conservation in proportion to the contribution of each to the total livestock unit usage. This system of recording is particularly applicable to enterprises receiving little additional feed while at grass.

A possible alternative to the livestock unit scheme involves using the actual liveweights of the recorded stock in place of the livestock unit values.

Forage crops

A whole range of crops can be grown in Britain to provide fresh vegetable matter for sheep feeding when grass is of poor quality or unavailable. These forage crops are usually integrated into the farming system, and will provide fresh material for feeding at any time from August to April according to the particular crop used. Two types of forage crop are used in Britain: those providing green leaves for sheep feeding and those that provide roots. The general characteristics of these crops vary considerably (Ingram, 1990), so careful matching of sheep requirements to crop characteristics is required (Table 5.10).

Green leaf crops
Forage crops grown for their leaves are usually from the brassica family and tend to be grown as catch crops providing feed in the autumn and early winter. Such catch crops are normally sown between June and August after the cereal harvest, before the ploughing of old pasture, or as part of a land reclamation programme, and they are grazed in situ.

Root crops
Forage crops of this type usually occupy the land for the whole growing season. They are therefore very expensive to grow and a high

Table 5.10 The feed characteristics of forage crops. (Source: Fitzgerald, 1983)

	Dry matter	Crude protein	Energy	Fibre	Digestibility
Green crops	Low	High	Moderate	Moderate	Moderate
Root leaves	Low	High	Low	Moderate	Moderate
Brassica roots	Very low	Moderate	High	Moderate	High
Beet roots	Variable	Low	Very high	Low	Very high

yield of material is required to justify the investment. Root crops are fed in late autumn and winter in situ, indoors or on grass.

Utilizing forage crops

Sheep should be introduced gradually to the forage crop over a period of about ten days with an adequate area of run back, preferably on to permanent pasture. The area of forage crop on offer at any one time should be controlled by folding, a fresh supply being offered where possible on a daily basis. The size of the fold should not be too large as this will allow the animals to walk through the crop picking out the youngest and most succulent portions and soiling the remainder, leading to high wastage. Sheep should not be forced to clear up soiled fodder as this will merely result in reduced growth rates.

As the season progresses, crop deterioration associated with leaf shedding and increasing fibre in the stems of leafy brassicas and frost damage in both leafy brassicas and swedes and turnips will lead to poorer crop utilization. The efficiency with which roots are utilized is also influenced by their degree of anchorage in the soil with varieties of poorly rooted Dutch turnips being particularly susceptible to a high degree of wastage.

Two examples of the levels of production that forage crops can support are shown in Tables 5.11 and 5.12 for rape and swedes respectively. These two tables show how crop yield, the efficiency of utilization, the type of lamb and the number of feeding days required affect the potential stocking rate. The additional factors which must

Table 5.11 Potential stocking rates for lambs on rape and soft turnips. (Source: Scottish Agricultural College)

Crop characteristics DM yield (t/ha)		3		4		5		6	
% utilization		50	70	50	70	50	70	50	70
Lamb type	Days feeding	Stocking rate (lambs/ha)							
Crossbred									
36 kg	45	33	47	44	63	55	79	67	95
32–35 kg	90	17	27	23	33	29	41	34	49
Hill									
28 kg	70	23	32	30	43	38	54	46	65

Table 5.12 Potential stocking rates for lambs on swedes. (Source: Scottish Agricultural College)

Crop yield (t/ha)	60	80	100
Lamb type	Stocking rate (lambs/ha)		
Crossbred			
70 days feeding	61	81	102
90 days feeding	47	63	79
Hill			
100 days feeding	44	59	73
130 days feeding	34	45	56

be considered when contemplating feeding forage crops are numerous and include the nutritive value of the feed, food conversion efficiency and intakes and the economics of using forage crops for lamb feeding.

The sheep enterprise in Britain is heavily dependent on good grassland management but well planned systems will also incorporate forage crops, arable by-products and concentrate feeds to get the most out of the flock. Despite the fact that these topics have been treated separately here, successful flock performance can only be achieved by the well planned integration of all these feeds. Their use must, of course, be cost effective: the extra production achieved from correct feeding must be worth more than the cost of achieving it.

Conserved forages

Hay, silage and straw can all be used as conserved feeds for sheep during the winter months when grazing and forage crops are either in short supply or provide inadequate levels of nutriments. The decision as to which type of conserved feed to use depends on a wide range of factors including the feed requirements of the ewe, the availability and cost of the feed, grassland management, the farming system and the availability and type of housing on the farm.

Whatever type of conservation is used for winter feeding, it is essential to have it analysed to give an indication of its nutritive value. Feed requirements during late pregnancy can be critical. Meeting these requirements without a knowledge of the composition of the ration is impossible and may prove very costly in terms of wasted feed or dead animals. In Britain there are several organizations which will undertake the analysis of feeds.

Hay and straw

The feeding value of hay is determined by the stage of growth of the herbage at cutting and by the losses which are incurred during the making. Both of these factors are reflected in the digestibility (D value) of the hay.

The potential intake of hay, straw and grass is also governed by its digestibility. Feed intake is directly related to the D value of the feed. Thus for a given level of production forages of high digestibility will be consumed in the greatest quantity and will require the least supplementation with compound feed, whereas forages of low digestibility will be consumed in smaller amounts and will require a higher level of supplementation.

Silage

The feeding value of silage is determined by the stage of growth of the herbage at cutting and by the ensiling process which follows. While the fall in D value of the original material undergoing a good fermentation could be expected to be only 1–2 units, the fall might be 3–4 units if it undergoes a butyric fermentation and as high as 10 units where extensive overheating takes place.

Whilst the potential intake of silage is governed by its particle length and digestibility, it can be reduced by the fermentation quality. For silage of a given digestibility, the highest intake (in terms of silage dry matter) can be expected where the herbage has been wilted to a dry matter of 25–28%, only a moderate level of acidity is present and it is relatively free from proteolysis. Potential intake will be reduced where the silage is wet and high in acid and will be lowest of all where the silage is wet and has a high degree of proteolysis. In general, only well wilted silages with a good fermentation should be used for sheep.

Concentrate feeds

Concentrate feeds are used in sheep production when the requirements of the ewes and lambs are high and the quality of the grazing or conserved feed is inadequate. Barley with a source of protein is the most common type of concentrate, although feed blocks are commonly used in some situations. Cereals in sheep diets are best fed as whole grains. This not only saves on processing costs but reduces the risk of acidosis. Protein sources such as soya bean meal, fish meal or some form of oilseed cake can supply enough protein for the ewes' needs at most times of the year.

Growing lambs on early weaning systems require access to high quality concentrate feeds in order to cash in on high growth rates and good early prices. Concentrates containing 18% crude protein in small pellets are ideal for weaned lambs.

Feed blocks are a convenient way of providing additional energy and protein in situations where herbage quality is poor and the ground is inaccessible. Although the intake of feed blocks may be low at certain times in the year, they make a valuable contribution to improving intake and efficiency. This effect is particularly beneficial when grazing quality is poor. Feed blocks are often expensive for the amount of energy they supply but they may prove economic in certain difficult conditions where no other options exist.

6 Fixed Resources

The fixed resources of a farming business are land, labour, capital and equipment, and the costs incurred by each of these are referred to as fixed costs. They cannot readily be allocated to any specific enterprise and will only alter significantly when substantial alterations to the business are made. The importance of any individual resource to the sheep enterprise depends on the nature of the enterprise, its location and its level of integration into the whole business. Fixed resources are often interdependent. For example, in hill or extensive production systems land is fixed and depends on adequate supplies of capital to exploit its full potential. Optimum output from stock resources depends on the full availability of the necessary feed and fixed resources.

The nature of fixed costs means that it is very dificult to make any kind of allocation to the sheep enterprise unless detailed whole farm recording is undertaken. MLC surveys of the fixed costs associated with sheep production in recorded lowland and upland flocks provide some information. These surveys, conducted over a three year period, show how costs may be allocated to the important fixed resources. Absolute financial figures are not presented as they bear little relation to the actual cost levels of production prevailing. However, the survey results do highlight the relative importance of each resource and show that the proportions were similar for both lowland and upland flocks (Table 6.1).

Labour costs, which are a significant proportion of total fixed costs, fall into two distinct groups: paid family labour and specialist shepherds. The element of family labour is more important in the upland flocks where over 60% of the total labour involvement is family as compared to just over 40% in lowland flocks. It was also established that a large proportion of labour input was allocated at lambing in both upland and lowland flocks (Table 6.2).

The limited time period covered by these surveys was insufficient to

Table 6.1 Structure of fixed costs in lowland and upland flocks (three year average). (Source: MLC, 1980b)

	Lowland (%)	Upland (%)
Rent and buildings	22	24
Machinery and equipment	18	17
Machinery running costs	6	6
Labour		
Paid	18	15
Family	21	28
Other fixed costs	14	12

Table 6.2 Structure of labour costs in lowland and upland flocks, 1977. (Source: MLC, 1980b)

	% labour costs	
	Lowland	Upland
Lambing	42	39
Rest of year	48	51
Conservation and forage	11	10

establish any major trends in fixed costs. However, it was possible to establish a close relationship between gross and net margins from those farms which were surveyed and also had the flock fully recorded by MLC. Thus gross and net margins could be calculated for a sample of flocks, and from this an analysis of the relationship between the two margins was also calculated. A large proportion of the variation in net margins per hectare (78%) was explained by the variation in gross margins per hectare. It is therefore reasonable to conclude that any factor influencing gross margins will also have an effect on net margins. The data supports the view that the gross margin of the sheep enterprise is a reliable indicator of profitability.

The fixed costs of the sheep enterprise are relatively low but it is difficult to obtain data to support this view. Whole farm data available from the Scottish Agricultural College provides some information on gross and net margins per hectare for some contrasting lowland enterprises (Table 6.3). Fixed costs associated with cereals

Table 6.3 Comparison of fixed costs per hectare (£). (Source: The Scottish Agricultural College, 1992)

	Cattle and sheep	Cereals	Dairy
Output	736	684	1818
Variable costs	290	251	717
Gross margin	446	433	1101
Fixed costs			
Labour	74	85	211
Machinery	127	131	264
Rent and rates	73	81	82
Others	68	79	184
Total	342	376	741
Net margin	104	57	360

and dairy farms are higher than those for cattle and sheep farms, with the result that the net margin per hectare is greatest for the latter.

Land

In a general livestock enterprise planning context the area of land available is almost always fixed, but because of modern technological advances in land improvement and utilization the output which can be obtained from this resource may be changed quite dramatically. In some cases the change may necessitate a complete revision of the enterprise plan.

The costs set against the enterprise reflect the rent charged for the area used, or the notional rent in the case of owner-occupied land. These rents reflect the production potential of the land, and if this is increased through improvement and capital investment then rents may go up. In extensive hill and upland areas improvements may involve land reclamation through fencing and reseeding, thereby increasing the stock carrying capacity of the area. Capital is required for the improvements themselves and also to purchase additional stock so that the sheep enterprise can expand and fully exploit the resources. In lowland areas improved drainage or the provision of irrigation will increase the potential of the land area, and if the sheep enterprise is not able to exploit these improvements then alternative enterprises could be sought. An example of enterprise substitution which occurred in Spain has already been discussed. In that case extensive grazing areas were improved through irrigation, but the increased grass supplies utilized by sheep could not compete with the margins available from cash crops grown on the same areas. The net result was the removal of the sheep enterprise from the improved ground to higher dry ground where the systems of production reverted to extensive management.

The value of a grazing livestock enterprise, and of sheep in particular, to the maintenance and development of the land resource is often ignored. Sheep provide valuable injections of fertility to the soil, the benefits of which are often not reaped until the sheep have been moved to a new area.

Labour

The people involved in the management of the flock are a critical component, and perhaps the major constraint to potential expansion or increased efficiency. The level of flock supervision varies depending on the availability of skilled labour and the intensity of production. Shepherding skills are an ever increasing expense to set against the output of the flock. Shepherds and their families are therefore being asked to take responsibility for increasingly larger flocks. In New Zealand, for example, one man is expected to look after on average 1500 ewes, backed up by gang labour at tailing, shearing and other key periods. The so called 'easy-care' sheep is the result.

Labour input in Britain falls into two important categories – paid family labour and specialized shepherds – which, as we have seen, together account for over 40% of the fixed costs of production in lowland and upland flocks. As these costs increase sheep producers are looking to contractual help for shearing, dipping and lambing. The creation of associations of sheep shearers and contractors in Britain reflects this trend.

Training in the routine tasks is essential. Shepherds are now asked to fulfil tasks such as condition scoring, lamb weighing and selection for slaughter over and above the more traditional management chores. Colleges provide valuable training for young entrants to the agricultural industry and a small number of colleges offer specialist courses in shepherding skills and flock management. Many specialist tasks cannot be taught, however, and are only learnt by experience.

An important element of the British sheep industry is the in-service training available to personnel in the industry under the auspices of several Agricultural Training Boards (ATB). ATB sponsored training groups around the country and specialist training courses are organized through a network of skilled training instructors from a wide spectrum of industry institutions.

Training in craft skills is an essential requirement for the labour involved with the flock, particularly as shepherds are increasingly asked to cut their labour involvement with the flock to a minimum. Routine tasks need to be completed more speedily.

Capital

Of the fixed resources, capital is arguably the most important. Land and labour cannot be fully exploited without access to funds, either in the form of working capital to meet the day to day needs of the enterprise or the much larger amounts of investment capital required to finance and run the business in the long term. Traditionally, sheep systems have been thought to have low capital requirements in Britain but, as more and more animals are stocked, sheep production is becoming increasingly capital intensive.

Comparisons with alternative enterprises indicate that peak working capital requirements of the ewe flock are as high or higher than some beef systems (Spedding, 1984). Estimated numbers of stock, gross margins and peak working capital on 20 ha of grass for three alternative beef systems and a ewe flock demonstrate the high capital requirements of the ewe flock relative to the gross margin (Table 6.4). These calculations relate to the establishment of each enterprise, and therefore with the ewe flock a significant proportion of the capital requirements relate to large once and for all payments for breeding stock purchases.

Working capital

Working capital is needed for an enterprise cycle, and for the sheep flock usually comprises livestock purchases and the variable costs of the enterprise. In the Flockplan scheme, working capital of the breeding ewe flock is defined as:

Table 6.4 Estimates of numbers of stock, annual gross margin and peak working capital for 20 ha. (Source: Spedding, 1984)

	Number of stock	Gross margin (£)	Peak working capital (£)
Ewe flock	262	7598	31356
Cereal beef	100	7900	38800
Silage beef	124	18228	43028
18-month beef	62	11532	29140
Dairying	40	18400	30000

- Valuation of the breeding stock in the flock
- Half the variable costs
- Flock replacement cost

The capital demands of the enterprise must be considered when assessing the viability or profitability of a new enterprise or reviewing the performance of an existing one.

An assessment of the movements of the funds involved in the enterprise over a defined period is given by the trading net cash flow. The cash flow per 100 ewes shown in Fig 6.1 identifies typical peak capital requirements. On mixed farms in Britain, the cash flow of the enterprise is probably less crucial than on farms where the sheep flock is the sole or major enterprise. However, in the mixed farm situation producers now consider the complementary nature of cash flows and the inter-relation of one with another. This can be illustrated by the following example. On a mixed farm with a large dairy herd as the main livestock enterprise and ware potatoes as the main arable crop, a large store lamb finishing unit can play an important role. The regular income from the dairy herd generates the cash flow to service the major items of fixed costs on the farm (rent and labour) while the complementary cash flows of the other two enterprises generate the real farm income. Cash returned from the ware potatoes in the mid-summer period is rolled into store lamb purchases which by the end of the winter period provide sufficient income to finance the new potato crop and release sufficient capital to provide the overall farm income.

An important item of working capital is the support element from subsidies which play an increasing role in the European sheep community. In Britain producers in hill and upland areas benefit from ewe subsidies paid under the Hill Livestock Compensatory Allowance

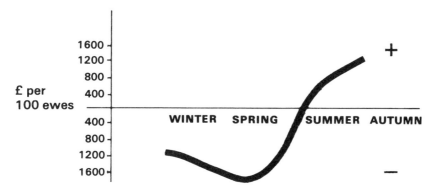

Fig. 6.1 Trading net cash flow for lowland flock

(HLCA) scheme. In addition to the direct support given to the sheep enterprise, this infusion of capital provides support to the general social structure of the agricultural community. In hill areas in particular this is vital as the majority of small village communities and associated urban centres depend on sheep farming for their survival.

Investment capital

Finance of this nature is long term, and before any large scale investments in the sheep enterprise are considered it is advisable to prepared detailed budgets for various alternatives. Capital investment for the sheep flock is normally associated with major items such as housing and handling equipment, aspects of land improvement such as fencing, drainage and reseeding. Justification for investment in these capital items is usually on the grounds of potential increase in output through improved labour efficiency or increased production from land resources.

An example of the financial benefits which can be achieved from capital investment in land improvement on a Welsh hill unit is available from Pwllpeiran EHF (Wildig, 1980). This financial evaluation showed that peak investment was reached at the end of the second year, and that the increased gross margin from the sheep and cattle enterprise had repaid the investment by the end of the sixth year and continued to benefit the unit at a high rate thereafter. Included in the investment were buildings, roads, silage machinery, costs of pasture improvement and additional fencing and livestock.

Housing and equipment

Labour involved with the flock is being asked to handle increasing numbers of ewes, and can only expect additional help at peak periods of the sheep year. Two items of fixed equipment can minimize the stress to both the labour and the sheep, and therefore allow more time and expertise to be devoted to the flock. The provision of semi-permanent winter housing is one of these major fixed items and the other involves some type of well designed sheep handling system.

Housing

An essential feature of many management systems in Europe is the winter housing of sheep. In Scandinavia, climatic conditions are such that ewes are confined throughout the winter months. In other European countries housing is less important although some breeds in France and Spain with extended breeding seasons, such as the Île de France, lamb in autumn and ewes remain housed through until spring. In the United States, large flocks in the Mid-west are housed for shelter from the low temperatures and high winds and protection against predators. Housing for variable periods over the winter has only recently become popular in Britain and the period of confinement varies widely within and between systems (Table 6.5).

A number of advantages are claimed for winter housing. Poaching, which delays spring growth and reduces total grass production, is almost eliminated with possible benefits in terms of higher summer stocking rates, while on arable farms grass leys can be ploughed up for

Table 6.5 Housing of ewes in Britain. (Source: MLC, Flockplan)

	System of production			
	Lowland		Upland	Hill
	Early lambing	Spring lambing		
Number of flocks	24	380	98	54
Percentage housing ewes	58	53	38	11
Average weeks housed	10	6	5	10
Average number of grazing days	190	192	181	174

autumn cereals. A major advantage to the shepherd managing the flock is that flock inspection and supervision at key times are eased, with resulting savings in lamb losses. Mortality of ewes may also be reduced and in extensive hill flocks housing can provide a less costly alternative to away wintering of ewes. However these advantages must, of course, be set against the disadvantages of high capital cost, increased maintenance costs and higher feed requirements.

Aspects of health in relation to the housing of ewes have been discussed in some detail by Linklater & Watson (1983). They point to the importance of building design, the provision of adequate ventilation and trough space, and the variety of flooring and bedding materials available.

Space does not permit detailed consideration of the housing of the ewe flock, but it is essential that anyone contemplating the erection of a winter sheep house should consult buildings advisers with experience of housed ewes.

Typical performance figures for a large lowland ewe flock for the year prior to housing and the five years following housing highlight the important benefits (Table 6.6). Ewes were housed from late January to after lambing. More lambs are born per 100 ewes mating and a greater portion are reared. The flock is stocked more intensively. The management and nutrition of the housed ewe requires particular attention if the marginally larger litters are not to be lost prior to lamb turn out. Many flockmasters who have introduced housing appear to have failed in exploiting its benefits.

The performance and management of housed ewes can be enhanced

Table 6.6 Performance of housed ewes. (Source: MLC, Flockplan)

	Year*				
	1	2	3	4	5
Total lambs born alive	100	103	102	108	110
Died after lambing	100	110	82	88	82
Number reared	100	101	102	109	109
Ewes/ha					
Summer	100	128	174	163	181
Grassland	100	142	168	170	189

* Indexed to 100 in year 1 when housing introduced.

through shearing just prior to housing. This allows stocking density to be marginally increased (by 5–10%) and permits easier inspection of body condition and udder development. Shorn ewes produce heavier, stronger lambs but inevitably eat more.

General guidelines on housing are available from the Farm Buildings Information Centre. Any sheep house should incorporate three important features: a dry bed, no draughts at animal level and air overhead, and adequate lying area. Provision of a dry bed can be achieved through straw bedding or slats, while animal penning to allow as much as 1.3 m^2/ewe and 500 mm of trough space per ewe is essential. A whole range of housing types from the most simple open yard to a complete off the shelf portal frame type of structure are available.

Planning the provision of winter housing for the flock requires careful thought. The capital cost of housing structures is the major consideration and will vary from type to type according to the method of construction, material used, etc. The advantages of each individual type must be weighed carefully. A rough guide to the comparative net costs for a range of different types is given in Table 6.7 where values are based on the cost of the most expensive palatial portal frame structure built by contractors. Expenditure on such a large capital and long term item can be considerable and mistakes expensive, so wherever possible the advice of specialists should be sought before a commitment to any one type is made.

Handling equipment

Provision of well designed handling equipment is an essential element of any well planned sheep unit. There are the obvious benefits to labour involved, and in addition many of the tasks necessary to achieve high levels of output demand good handling facilities. Pen

Table 6.7 Housing cost relative to the most expensive portal frame building. (Source: Farm Buildings Information Centre)

Topless yard	7–13
Plastic tunnel	17
New monopitch with partly covered yard	22
Second-hand farm built portal frame	27
Farm built portal frame	40
Basic portal by contractors	67
Palatial portal by contractors	100

layouts are often dictated by the sites and vary from farm to farm. Planning and forethought are required before any new installations are provided.

The exact requirements will depend on the size of the flock and the geography of the site. Certainly there is no single standard layout which is suitable for every flock, but some general points can be made. Firstly, it is preferable if the unit chosen is relatively inexpensive and simple to build. It must also be simple to operate and maintain over a long period. Units should be placed as close to the sheep grazing areas as possible, with access to good services. A well drained and sheltered site should always be the aim.

Basic design requirements must include three areas: one for gathering sheep, one for working and a third for holding or drafting. Consideration should be given to the shape of gathering pens, gate entrances and race angles to encourage animals to move freely in the system. Working areas should encompass small handling and treatment pens, drafting and shedding arrangements, and footbath and dipping facilities. In the overall general design consideration should also be given to other features which are required such as entry to a weigh crate, access for loading and unloading, and shearing facilities.

The assimilation of all the requirements of the handling system and full incorporation into a workable fixture on the farm requires skill and knowledge. Assistance from a specialist with all this information and experience at his fingertips is always recommended.

7 Exploiting Resources

The exploitation of resources for sheep production does not necessarily stop at farm level. There are many instances around the world where the organization of sectors of the national sheep industry can lead to an improved exploitation of resources. These industry structures rarely encompass the whole of a country's sheep industry and several different industry structures may be apparent in one country, ranging in size from a group of cooperating farms to a significant proportion of the national breeding flock.

Industry structures around the world are seldom the result of a national plan. More often they reflect the optimum production from animal resources through the manipulation of feed and fixed resources. This is generally achieved through the ingenuity of the individual farm manager to exploit and utilize the biological characteristics of his sheep and other resources. An awareness and understanding of the more common structures is central to any improvement plan.

It is important to remember that within any industry many factors, which have a direct bearing on the decision making process and the product, are to some degree fixed. It is the manipulation of those factors which are not fixed that allows industry structures to develop. Current industry structures should not be regarded as static but merely as a reflection of the present way of things. Three major types of industry structures can be identified: self-contained purebreeding, self-contained pure and crossbreeding, and cross-breeding.

Purebreeding

Industry structures based on purebreeding are characterized by breeds which produce all their own replacements and where the production objectives of the sector are all met from one type of ewe. Many such industry structures involve large purebred flocks which are self replacing on the ewe side and which may or may not buy in rams from elsewhere. These flocks are a common feature of extensive sheep keeping areas, of which Australia, New Zealand and South Africa are good examples. Flocks of this type are also widely distributed around Europe. They have certain advantages because of the simple breeding objectives and plans can be drawn up to a fairly rigid pattern without the added complications which are introduced when crossing is involved.

Purebred flocks are commonly associated with wool production although many examples can be found in Europe where meat production is the primary objective. In Holland, for example, the Texel breed is maintained purely for its meat production while in Britain, where crossbreeding is the most common feature, large self-contained flocks of hill ewes are maintained, notably of the Scottish Blackface, Welsh Mountain and Swaledale breeds.

In a number of instances purebred performance has been insufficient for the requirements of the market, and new breeds have been created through organized crossbreeding. In this way increased ewe bodyweights, fertility and wool yields have been achieved. However, once this step forward was achieved the illusion of new blood ceased and the previous policies of within flock selection and improvement were re-adopted. This practice has been widespread in New Zealand, South America and South Africa, with the result that large populations of Merino and Romney stocks have been replaced with various improved wool-producing breeds such as Coopworth and Corriedales in New Zealand, the Dohne Merino in South Africa and the Columbia in the Americas.

Within flock selection is also considerably more straightforward for purebred flocks, particularly with wool traits. Fleece weights and quality are moderately heritable characters. Measurements taken within the flock and the selection of ewe and ram replacements on the basis of this information can prove beneficial. However, in breeds where sheepmeat is the primary product and reproductive performance, carcase weight and carcase quality are the important components of production, within flock selection is therefore more complicated.

Self-contained pure and crossbreeding

A number of industry structures rely on large self-contained purebred flocks in which surplus breeding females are mated to rams of another

breed. These are generally dual-purpose breeds exploiting the purchased ewes for one particular product, i.e. wool or milk. Crossing the
ewes with a terminal sire breed gives lambs more suited to carcase
production. Structures such as these tend to be fragmented, especially
where differing climates, product preferences and terminal sire breeds
exist. However, improvement within the self-contained pure breed is
straightforward for the primary product though little direct
improvement can be applied to the secondary product. Producers
have to be selective in the choice of crossing ram and therefore must
rely on the appropriate improvements to be made in the purebred
flocks from which rams are chosen.

Numerous examples of this type of structure exist around the world.
In France, for example, there are many self-contained purebred flocks
in which a significant proportion of the ewes are mated to rams from
breeds with good carcase characteristics, e.g. Charollais. The carcases
produced from this cross are more valuable than those produced pure
within the flock. This mixture of purebreeding and crossbreeding is
also a feature of many large flocks in central Europe, mainly of the
Merino type. These flocks are primarily kept for the production of
large quantities of fine wool but, again, a proportion of the ewes are
mated to terminal sires with improved carcase characteristics. The
lamb carcases produced are then available for export to Italy or the
Middle East.

Crossbreeding in the Manchega dairy flocks in Spain has led to a
marked increase in output per ewe and overall efficiency. The average
carcase weight produced was increased from 10 kg to 18 kg by crossing
surplus ewes to a terminal sire breed. A similar situation is found in
French dairy breeds where the best milking ewes are bred pure to elite
tested rams. These matings produce the female replacements for the
milking flock. Young ewes and those considered to have inferior
performance are mated to terminal sires for meat production.

A further attempt to utilize this mixed type of structure has been set
up by the US Feed Grains Council in the Mediterranean area. The
main objective of the new structure has been to utilize grains as a feed
source in an area where, traditionally, they have not been exploited.
Local ewes kept under extensive systems have been mated to rams of
the meat breeds and the resulting lambs have been moved to intensive
feedlots for finishing at a much earlier age than normal, i.e. three to six
months rather than the traditional one to three years. This approach
has been successful in countries such as Syria where additional

benefits to those already mentioned have been achieved through the release of feed resources for the breeding ewes.

Crossbreeding

This final group of industry structures exploit crossbreeding to its fullest extent and are characterized by ewes being moved from one location to a second for crossing with rams of another breed.

Crossbreeding is generally associated with meat production. The two biological components which affect the efficiency of meat production are the reproductive performance of the ewe and the growth and carcase characteristics of the lamb. It is considered appropriate in a breeding programme to exploit the ewe reproductive aspects in a female line and exploit the growth and carcase potential in the sire breed of the lamb. Improvement of ewe reproductive performance is always considered to be slow (although it is perfectly feasible) and many ideas are put forward to increase reproductive performance, in particular lambing performance, with a crossbred ewe derived from highly prolific types. The Finnish Landrace and Romanov breeds have been widely employed in the production of crossbred ewes for this purpose, with varied success.

Systematic crossbreeding is a key feature of the British system of sheep production which is unlike the national industry of any other country. The stratified sheep industry in Britain is widely cited as a valuable structure which exploits the wide range of farm environments for meat production and its complexities and individuality warrant detailed consideration. Many visitors to Britain are quite naturally confused by the changing nature of the flocks as they drive around the countryside. Within a short distance, quite distinct flock types can be seen.

The industry is characterized by a stratified three-tier breeding structure related to the altitude and quality of grazing. The first tier is in the hill areas where ewes of the hill breeds, of which the Scottish Blackface, Welsh Mountain and Swaledale are the most numerous, are maintained in self-contained flocks under the relatively harsh environments of the hills and mountains (700–1000 m). Surplus breeding stock from these flocks in the form of cast-for-age ewes are transferred into the uplands, the second tier of the industry, where they are crossed with specialized longwool ram breeds such as the

Bluefaced Leicester and the Border Leicester. Conditions are generally kinder in these areas. The first-cross ewe lambs produced here are transferred to the lowland areas which represent the third tier of the structure (Fig. 7.1). Crossbred ewe flocks in the lowlands produce a significant proportion of the total sheepmeat. Here ewes are generally crossed with rams of the terminal sire breeds to produce slaughter lambs.

The net result is that systematic crossbreeding is a key feature of the British system of sheep production and that a high proportion of the sheepmeat produced is derived from crossbred lambs. However, there are exceptions to this generalized crossbreeding structure since within the upland and lowland sectors of the industry self-contained flocks are also found. The stratified system has not always been a feature of British sheep farming but is a recent development arising out of the general upheaval during the period of the 1914–18 war. At that time many pastures were ploughed up to provide additional arable cash crops as part of the war effort. In the period immediately after the war these became an embarrassment and large tracts were returned to grass. However, over that period the large Down flocks which had been found throughout central and southern England were under-

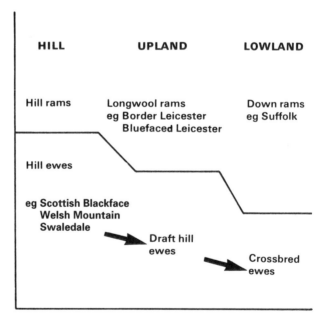

Fig. 7.1 Three-tier structure of sheep production in Britain. (Source: MLC, 1988b)

going a marked decline in population so that when large areas of ground were returned to grass in the aftermath of the war lowland stock numbers were extremely low. The major source of stock then became the hill and upland regions and large numbers of sheep were brought in from these areas, probably in the form of draft ewes at first and then later as crossbred ewes. In the years between the wars low input farming was widely practised in the midlands of England as the general economy stagnated, and the link between lowland and hill areas became established.

A clearer picture of the industry was provided by two MLC surveys completed in 1972 and 1987, the results of which provided a more detailed description of the stratified crossbreeding system and identified over seventy pure breeds and 300 crossbred types (MLC, 1988b). These results reveal a small number of breeds which have a considerable influence within the industry, either by their numerical dominance or through their use in crossbreeding. They are:

Hill
    Scottish Blackface
    Welsh Mountain
    North Country Cheviot
    Swaledale
Longwool
    Bluefaced Leicester
    Border Leicester
Down
    Suffolk

Together, these purebreds account for over 35% of the total ewe population, and the crossbred ewes derived from them account for a further 40%. The most comprehensive description of these breeds and the large number of other British breeds can be found in *British Sheep* (National Sheep Association, 1992).

The generalized structure of the industry outlined earlier was demonstrated by the 1987 survey to be an oversimplification. The pattern of pure and crossbreeding was more fragmented than had been thought and a number of regional variations on the general crossbreeding theme were revealed. For example, a high proportion of draft hill ewes in Wales were mated directly to a Down ram for slaughter lamb production, a practice which accounted for almost half the matings of draft hill ewes maintained in the uplands areas.

Regional variation between Scotland and northern England was found in the production of crossbred ewes for sale to the lowland areas. In northern England nearly all the crossbred ewe lambs out of the Cheviot and Swaledale hill ewes were retained and subsequently mated to Down rams on lowland farms. By contrast, in Scotland only about 15% of the Border Leicester × Blackface ewe lambs were kept for breeding. The important variations are summarized in Fig. 7.2.

The systematic crossbreeding system has considerable merit as a method of adapting sheep production to a range of farm environments. Extensive areas of mountain and hill are utilized by the large population of hill ewe breeds. The production of crossbred ewes from these hill breeds by crossing with a specialized Longwool ram results in a ewe which has a higher prolificacy and bodyweight than its purebred mother, and in addition offers the likelihood of beneficial maternal heterosis. The use of the terminal meat-sire breed on the crossbred ewe provides the means to tailor the slaughter lamb carcase to meet the requirements of the market.

It is therefore possible within this crossbreeding system for producers to plan the optimum production from the animal resources at their disposal in order to meet the needs of the market. However, it is difficult to ensure a general balance between the production of crossbred ewes and the demand from lowland flockmasters for them as replacements. A weakness of the system is the possibility of short-term supply problems which can distort ewe prices. These fluctuations may be of greater concern to the supplier in the hills than the lowland buyer as the price received for these breeding ewes forms a major part of his income. A further weakness of the system is that regular transfer of breeding stock increases the risk of spreading disease. Deaths from sporadic disease outbreaks such as infectious abortion can cause serious loss and disruption to the lowland flock.

The crossbreeding structure of the British sheep industry evolved due to economic and social pressures during the early part of the twentieth century. Other crossbreeding structures have been set up specifically to exploit certain genetic characteristics found in particular breeds. In France, for example, an attempt has been made to produce a more prolific female by crossing French breeds with the highly prolific Romanov breed from northern Europe. The resulting first cross (F_1) females are then mated to a terminal sire for lamb carcase production. Originally this system was developed using rams of the Romanov breed mated to local ewes. This produced the required F_1 females but the system had to carry the burden of the less

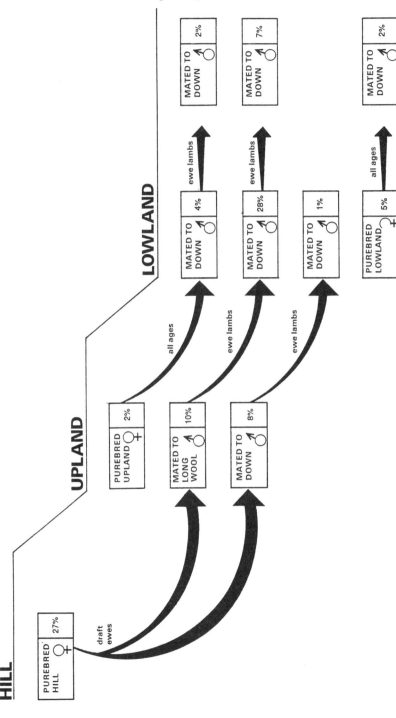

Fig. 7.2 Main components of breeding structure. (Source: MLC, 1988b)

productive local sheep at some extra cost. A more productive system is now being exploited by crossing local rams with Romanov ewes. While this does not alter the production potential of the F_1 females, the system as a whole is more productive due to the better rearing performance found in the Romanov ewe.

It is interesting to compare the original French system, i.e. prolific ram crossed with local breed of ewe, with its equivalent in the British system. While in the French system the low level of performance of the ewe from the local breed was considered a drawback, this is not the case in Britain. The local breed in Britain, the draft hill ewe, is kept in an environment where a lower level of performance is acceptable as the system is of the low-input/low-output type. In France the local ewe breed is kept under much the same conditions as the F_1 and thus incurs a level of cost which its performance cannot justify.

Section 3
Production Systems

In this section an attempt is made to show how the resources described in Section 2 are combined into viable production systems in Britain. The section is divided into three chapters dealing with hill, upland and lowland production systems. The division of systems in this way is somewhat arbitrary in that no physical boundaries exist between the

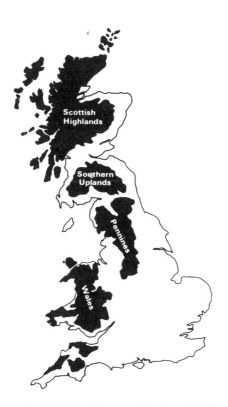

Hill and upland areas in Britain. (Source: Hughes, 1976)

three defined areas. For the purposes of this section, systems are grouped according to the level of ewe subsidy received under the Less Favoured Areas Directive of the EC. Hill systems contain ewes receiving the higher level of subsidy, upland systems contain ewes receiving the lower rate of subsidy and lowland systems are the remainder. The uplands and hills are shown as dark shaded areas and the lowlands are the unshaded areas in the map.

Upland flocks have similar output to lowland flocks but achieve this with lower costs and returns.

The profitability of hill flocks is much less than that of the other two types even though a much lower level of costs is incurred for production. The most noticeable feature of the comparison in the table is the contribution that subsidies make to output in the hill and upland areas. This is a particular feature of sheep production in these regions.

Throughout this section a range of production systems are discussed. In order to emphasize the value of comparative physical and financial data to the analysis and planning of an enterprise, results for typical flocks are compared with the relevant target performance of each system.

The relative economic performance of lowland, upland and hill systems in the UK. (Source: MLC, 1990)

	Upland*	Hill
Lamb sales	88	40
Wool sales	81	64
Ewe subsidies	172	221
Output	98	74
Total variable costs	77	44
Gross margin per ewe	110	92
Gross margin per hectare	90	—

* Values indexed to lowland performance = 100

8 Hill Sheep Production

Hill pastures occupy a major proportion of the land devoted to agricultural use in the UK. Although it is difficult to obtain precise information on the actual area involved in hill sheep production, it has been estimated that hill sheep farming and upland rearing farms account for a third of all UK farm land (EDCA, 1973). Of this area some 70% is unimproved natural grassland. The production of sheep from these hill areas is by far the most common farm enterprise. MAFF (1977) shows that 100% of hill farms in Britain keep breeding ewes, and these ewes constitute 43% of all ewes kept in the United Kingdom.

Although sheep production is a very important part of land use in hill areas, it is in direct competition with forestry, tourism, conservation and water storage and there are thus alternative demands on hill grazing land. Nevertheless the position of hill sheep in the structure of the UK industry is very important and, as has been shown in Chapter 7, the hills provide an abundant supply of breeding ewes for use in other sectors of the industry.

The principle features of sheep production in hill areas are low reproductive performance associated with the inadequacy of the nutrition provided by the natural grazings, and prolonged growth and development in the lambs produced. Despite these low levels of productivity and pressures from the forestry industry, there has been a dramatic increase in the numbers of hill ewes since the early 1970s. Ewe subsidies provided under the Less Favoured Areas Directive, the general buoyant nature of the whole industry in the eighties and the introduction of the EC Sheepmeat Regime are the main reasons.

The evolution of breeding ewe numbers over the past twenty years highlights a large increase in ewe numbers overall, and a most dramatic increase in England and Wales where the hill ewe population has risen by over 56% and 57% respectively since 1971 (Table 8.1). A large proportion of family farms with a supply of family labour and

Table 8.1 Hill ewe numbers 1971 to 1991 (000 head). (Source: MAFF)

	1971	1991	% increase
England	1175	1828	56
Wales	1620	2552	57
Scotland	2291	2312	< 1

land more suitable for improvement are two possible reasons for this expansion in Wales. In Scotland, on the other hand, ewe numbers have remained almost static due to the presence of larger estate farms, the greater distances to primary markets for lamb and the lower availability of labour.

Hill ewes utilizing the extensive areas of hill grazings provide three main products: lambs for feeding or slaughter, draft ewes and wool. There is also a significant amount of direct ewe subsidy which makes a fourth contribution to farm incomes and can therefore be considered along with the main products. Results from the Flockplan scheme demonstrating the relative contribution of the four components of gross output are shown in Fig. 8.1. Income from lambs, wool and draft ewes forms the major part, totalling 70% of gross output. The magnitude of the subsidy element may seem surprising but it must be remembered that maintenance of a viable livestock industry in the hill

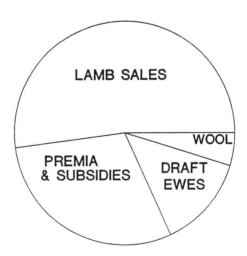

Fig. 8.1 Factors contributing to gross output in recorded hill flocks in 1989. (Source: MLC, 1990)

sector is vital if the social structure of the remoter areas is to remain intact and rural depopulation be avoided. The increasing role of the subsidy element in British hill sheep production cannot be ignored. In 1993, LFA payments and ewe premia together amounted to around 40% of gross receipts of the average hill flock.

The profitability of hill flocks is much more dependent upon climatic variation from year to year than that of upland and lowland flocks, although the injection of capital into hill areas can go some way towards reducing these effects. The ewe herself is the most important element in such systems and to some extent acts as a buffer to both the variable climate and the quality of grazing. Good hill ewes must conceive regularly, be able to produce an adequate milk supply and confer a good growth rate on their lambs under these difficult conditions. This should ensure that a good crop of lambs are born, suckle well and then survive the first critical days of life on the open hill.

Under traditional systems of management, however, performance levels are variable, mainly as a result of inadequate nutrition at critical periods of the year. These are recognized as the premating period, the last six to eight weeks of pregnancy when foetal growth is increasing rapidly, early lactation, and, for those ewes rearing twins, the lactation period.

Increased output from hill flocks can be achieved through careful planning of the allocation of the available nutrients, which in turn depends to a large extent upon land improvement.

Resources

The resources available to the flockmaster in hill situations are less flexible than those in other sectors of the industry. Traditional hill sheep farms have self-replenishing flocks with ewes kept in regular ages, and in most instances ewe stocks remain when ownership or tenancy of the land is changed. There is thus little movement of ewe stock between hill flocks, and any major changes are brought about by the introduction of rams. Traditionally, flocks are purebred but in a small proportion crossbreeding is practised. Away wintering of ewe replacements, known as agistment or tack, on lowland grass farms is a common feature in hill areas but increased rental charges have caused some producers to reconsider this practice and maintain the animals on their own farm. The physical characteristics of the common hill breeds are small body size and coarse fleece. The Scottish Blackface and Swaledale are horned, while the Welsh Mountain and Hill Cheviot breeds are polled. Another feature of these ewes is low productivity. Weaning percentages can vary widely from around 60 up to 120 on the better hill farms. Weaning weights of individual animals also vary, reflecting the quality of the hill grazings available.

Results from MLC recorded flocks over the period 1985–89 (Table 8.2) show the levels of profitability in hill flocks at that time and the annual variation encountered in some physical parameters. More recently, although margins have remained the same, the proportion of price support is greater. However, with severe financial constraints on hill flocks, few flocks can afford to record, therefore the MLC database is now quite limited for this sector.

Production data from two hill flocks on the Ministry of Agriculture, Fisheries and Food (MAFF) Experimental Husbandry Farm (EHF) at Pwllpeiran illustrates the low performance levels observed in Welsh Mountain hill flocks (Table 8.3).

Table 8.2 Results from hill flocks 1985–89. (Source: MLC, 1990)

	1985	1986	1987	1988	1989
Net output (£/ewe)	38.9	42.8	46.0	44.6	41.0
Total variable costs (£/ewe)	9.3	10.6	10.5	9.1	9.0
Gross margin (£/ewe)	29.6	32.2	35.5	35.5	32.0
No. lambs reared per ewe	1.05	1.02	1.08	1.09	1.07
Finished lambs sold/100 ewes mated	20	19	20	28	30

Table 8.3 Production data for two hill flocks of Welsh Mountain ewes: three year means. (Source: Wildig, Richards & Roberts, 1982)

	Tynbryn unit	Blaenmyherin unit
Pre-mating ewe weight (kg)	33	34
Wool weight (kg)	1.6	1.6
Weaning percentage	95	102
Lamb weight at 18 weeks (kg)	20.6	22.3
Ewes per hectare	1.51	2.41
Ewe replacement weights (kg)		
at 7 months	22	23
at 12 months	26	28

Table 8.4 Physical performance levels in recorded hill flocks, 1989. (Source: MLC, 1990)

	Average	Top third*
Flock size	918	776
Ewes lambing (%)	94	95
No. of lambs born per ewe mated	111	124
No. of lambs reared per ewe mated	107	122
Lambs retained for breeding (% of lambs reared)	36	42
Lambs sold finished (% of lambs reared)	28	27

* Top third selected on gross margin per ewe

Physical performance data from average and top third flocks recorded by MLC in 1989 (Table 8.4) illustrate the productive characteristics of hill sheep and the variability of these characters in the hill environment.

These levels of individual animal performance are well below the known genetic potential of hill sheep. Draft ewes moved to lower and more producitve pastures show a marked increase in weaning percentage and this response is exploited by producers within the industry. Lamb growth rate is also severely depressed under hill conditions yet if Scottish Blackface lambs are fed intensively gains in excess of 300 g/day can be demonstrated, in marked contrast to the average gains under normal hill conditions of around 150 g/day.

Low reproductive performance, poor lamb growth, high mortality of ewes and lambs and low stocking rates are linked to the poor nutritional supplies of hill pastures. Work at the Hill Farming Research Organisation (HFRO) indicates that the reproductive potential of most hill breeds is severely depressed by nutrition under hill conditions. Increases in animal output depend on the improved availability of feed resources and this in turn requires investment in land and pasture improvement.

Feed resources available to the ewe flock consist mainly of the rough grazings which predominate on hill farms (around 95% of the land falls into that category). These grazings are variable, with the size and distribution of different types of vegetation influencing the nutritional supplies available to the ewes and the prospects for any possible improvements. The production potential of these hill pastures depends on factors such as soil type, moisture level or drainage characteristics, soil pH, phosphate, potash and nitrogen, most of which are limiting to some degree. There is a wide diversity between farms and even variation on a single hillside for these factors.

Traditionally, hill sheep are set stocked in a free grazing system and are expected to obtain most of their nutrient requirements from grazed pastures throughout the year, although supplementary feeding is increasingly being used. Grazing management practices vary widely from maintaining 'hefts' or 'cuts' (sub-flocks habitually grazing within the confines of a particular area of ground) to daily routine movements of ewes to the lower ground during the day and the higher ground in the late afternoon – a method known as 'raking'. Stocking rate is low – from 0.75–4.0 ha/ewe – and is determined by the winter carrying capacity of the hill. Variations in winter management occur in Wales where the sheep are moved into enclosed paddocks or 'ffridd' on the lower hill and in the north-east of Scotland where forage crops, mainly roots, are used as part of the winter feed. On many hill farms there will be an enclosed area adjacent to the steading, referred to as in-bye land, which is often the only source of conserved fodder.

Increasing output from hill flocks

The key to increased production in hill flocks is land improvement. This provides better quality pasture during lactation and improvements can be made to lamb growth rates, ewe bodyweight recovery and conception rates in the late summer and autumn. The planned management of these improved resources can lead to considerable increases in the total weight of saleable lamb obtained from the hill flock and thereby increase total flock output. Several methods for land improvement are available but factors such as soil type, existing vegetation, access and capital availability will all influence the choice of techniques adopted.

The fastest response can be achieved through mechanical cultivation, ploughing or rotavation and the reseeding of suitable level areas. Although this is one of the costliest techniques it can be made cheaper through the use of pioneer crops such as rape or stubble turnips for a store lamb fattening enterprise, prior to sowing down with grass. These techniques have been particularly successful at the Redesdale EHF.

An alternative and cheaper method is simply to fence suitable areas, apply lime and phosphate and use the grazing animal to control vegetation at key times. On pastures dominated by purple moor grass

(*Molinia caerulea*) improvements have been achieved by fencing, applying lime and phosphate, stocking heavily to remove surplus vegetation and broadcasting grass and clover seed.

Wherever pasture improvement is implemented, grass growth must be controlled with the grazing animal in order to prevent the influx of less productive species and the reversion to unimproved pasture. The grazing management of improved pasture is therefore critical.

Two pasture system

The integration of improved hill ground and tracts of unimproved hill has been demonstrated as a practical and effective means of increasing output from the hill flock. This method, known as the 'two pasture system', utilizes the improved areas for grazing the lactating ewes and during the premating period (Fig. 8.2).

After mating, all the ewes are wintered on the open hill pasture. Hay is fed if the natural vegetation is in short supply or covered by snow. Feed blocks are provided for ewes on the hill at least ten weeks before lambing starts (one 25 kg block per thirty ewes per week). If concentrates are fed these should be made on an increasing scale from 250 g per ewe per day six weeks before lambing to 500 g per day at lambing. If possible, two-year-old and lean ewes are drawn from February onwards, moved to improved pasture and fed at twice these levels.

Lambing takes place in enclosures, whenever possible, to allow some supervision. This need not be on an improved area – a cheaply fenced hill block is adequate – and this then allows the improved ground to make some growth. Lactating ewes are afterwards moved to

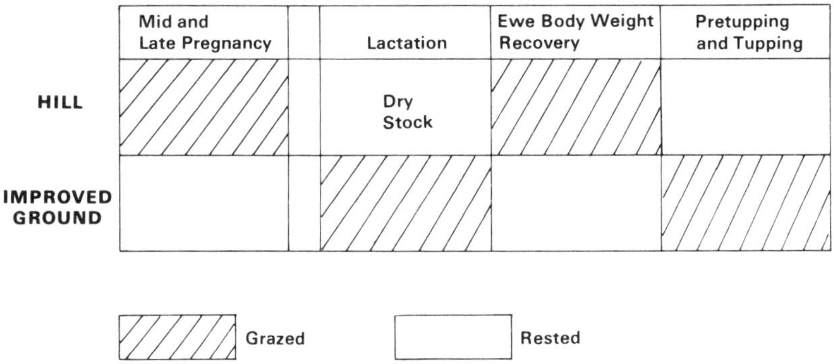

	Mid and Late Pregnancy		Lactation	Ewe Body Weight Recovery	Pretupping and Tupping
HILL	/////		Dry Stock	/////	
IMPROVED GROUND			/////		/////

///// Grazed   Rested

Fig. 8.2 Two pasture system. (Source: HFRO)

improved ground to graze for a week or more, the aim being to establish strong, well-grown lambs.

The area of improved ground determines the numbers that can utilize it, and ewes with twins are always given priority. If sufficient grazing is available the younger ewes with singles may also be grazed on the improved ground. The hill ground is used by all dry stock and all those singles which cannot be accommodated on better pasture. At weaning, lambs are sold or moved to hay aftermaths on the in-bye ground and the ewes returned to the open hill. The improved ground is then rested to allow regrowth.

The ewes are brought down on to the rested grass ground a month or so before tupping to maintain or improve their body condition. Ideally, sufficient improved grazing should be available to carry the ewes through at least the first cycle of mating, after which they can be returned to the hill to complete mating.

The principles of the system can be applied to most hill farms but the way in which they are followed will be determined by individual farm circumstances. On Agrostis-Festuca pastures, for instance, enough improved ground could be created to carry all nursing ewes but it is unlikely that it would be financially worthwhile to reseed enough ground to carry all ewes through lactation.

The system has been developed at a number of sites and the two examples which follow illustrate the benefits in terms of increased performance and output.

Example 1:
Sourhope, Hill Farming Research Organisation (283 ha) – North Country Cheviot × South Country Cheviot ewes

---

Over a five year period beginning in 1968, five 20 ha areas of Agrostis-Festuca pasture were enclosed by fencing. No lime or slag was applied until 1973. These areas have been used by ewes with singles. Twin-nursing ewes were grazed on the in-bye pasture until 1974 when reseeded areas were created for twins.

The numbers of ewes carried on this block of land were almost doubled and individual animal performance was significantly improved (Table 8.5).

Example 2:
Redesdale Experimental Husbandry Farm, Northumberland – Scottish Blackface ewes

---

Table 8.5 Results for the two pasture system at Sourhope. (Source: Armstrong, Eadie & Maxwell, 1978)

	Year 1	Year 3	Year 6	Year 8
No. of ewes	398	518	600	620
Weaning %	85	103	92	109
Weaning weight av. (kg)	22.6	26.7	26.1	26.6
Total weight of weaned lamb (kg)	7924	14177	14329	17902

In 1968, on a Molinia (purple moor grass) dominant sward, approximately 15% of the area was fenced, limed and slagged. The area was heavily stocked with cattle to remove rough vegetation and was then oversown with a clover/grass mixture the following year.

After ten years, the stock carrying capacity of the hill was doubled and individual animal performance increased significantly (Table 8.6).

An initial investment of capital is required to create the improved ground and extra capital investment will be involved as more breeding stock are retained. When considering the system care should be taken that the expected improvement in output will be sufficient to meet any annual charge on borrowed money.

Once the system is operating it will normally generate capital for carrying out further improvement work. As more and more improved ground is created, it is possible that other enterprises could make use of some of it once the requirements of the hill flock have been met. Extra conservation ground is invariably at a premium on hill land and would create more aftermath grazing for weaned lambs. Alternatively,

Table 8.6 Results from the two-pasture system at Redesdale EHF. (Source: MAFF, 1980)

	Year 1	Year 3	Year 8	Year 10
No. of ewes	155	224	317	372
Weaning %	73	99	114	91
Weaning weight (kg)	27.4	31.3	32.8	33.4
Total weight of weaned lamb (kg)	3095	6883	10909	10889

the land could be used for cattle grazing or as an area for an alternative flock of larger, more productive ewes.

Twin splitting

Increased proportions of twin lambs born in hill flocks, mainly as a result of improved nutrition at the critical periods, can present some management problems. Through the early weaning of one twin lamb from a pair and the return of the other to the hill with the ewe, two good lambs can be produced at the end of the summer. This contrasts with the usual situation of two twins of low bodyweight having a low value in the store market. The technique of twin splitting has received some attention in recent years and is now regarded as a viable proposition which makes use of a minimum area of improved pasture and makes maximum use of hill grazing.

In EHF trials early weaned lambs stocked at fifty to the hectare grew at an acceptable rate, while unweaned lambs achieved performance levels equivalent to those of single lambs reared under hill conditions. Where the twins are of mixed sexes the male lamb is weaned, and where they are of equal sexes the smaller of the two lambs should be weaned. Results from Redesdale EHF (Table 8.7) demonstrate the weights achieved for hill reared and early weaned twins. These results indicate that the hill reared lambs grew faster but would be subject to a later weaning check. This is borne out by similar work at Liscombe EHF where the weight comparison was followed through to November with Welsh Halfbred lambs. At this final stage weights were very similar for the two groups.

Table 8.7 Twin splitting. (Source: MAFF, 1981b)

	Average weight (kg)	
	Splitting early June	End August
Ewe		
Hill reared	14.8	30.4
Early weaned	13.9	27.7
Ram		
Hill reared	15.8	32.5
Early weaned	15.5	29.0

Indoor finishing of lambs

A recent development aimed at improving the income from hill flocks involves the indoor finishing of small hill lambs. These lambs may only be about 25 kg in weight in the autumn and would normally be sold as store lambs for little value. However, by housing the lambs and feeding them on concentrates and hay it is possible to sell them as finished lambs at 37 kg in weight. A typical budget for the finishing of hill lambs is summarized in Table 8.8. These figures indicate a useful source of additional income for hill farmers, although care must be taken when making the transition from a grazed diet to the concentrate diet.

Real-time scanning

The technique of real-time scanning described in Chapter 4 appears to be especially valuable to the hill farmer on improved land where a 10–20% twinning rate is expected. The accurate detection of foetal numbers can be beneficial in terms of improved foetal growth, resulting in lower lamb mortality, a clear identification of barren ewes with obvious cost savings and generally improved flock management. The ability to organize the grazing management of the flock before the lamb crop is delivered is a powerful tool.

Table 8.8 The economics of finishing hill lambs indoors, winter 1993. (Source: Scottish Agricultural College, 1992)

	£ per lamb
Output	
Lamb sales	31.65
Less lamb value at start	15.00
Feeders margin	16.65
Input	
Concentrates (80.0 kg)	9.20
Hay (15 kg)	0.10
Other costs	3.00
Total variable costs	12.30
Gross margin	4.35

Resource management

Capital investment in pasture improvement which increases the availability of feed resources creates a need for a careful flock management strategy. The return on investments in hill flocks is limited and therefore new investments must be fully cost effective to be justified. Although the detailed nature of these plans will vary according to the individual farm situation, it is worth discussing an example in detail to crystalize some of the critical components of these enterprises.

In the hill areas of Wales, mountain pastures are found in conjunction with enclosed paddocks on the lower part of the hill. Land improvement on the open hill creates a third manageable feed resource which then releases some of the grazing pressure from these ffridd and enables their production capabilities to be exploited more fully. Management in this type of situation has been an area of work at Pwllpeiran EHF and a summary of their management recommendations demonstrates how the integration of separate feed resources for the flock exploits each to its full potential (Table 8.9).

Under this system of management ewe weights, lamb weights and lambing percentages are significantly higher than in conventionally managed flocks where no improved mountain pastures are available. The improved pasture enables ewes and lambs to be sent to the mountain three to four weeks earlier than was previously possible. This means conservation areas can be closed earlier, and a small acreage can be released to grow forage crops for fattening wether lambs if required. Pressure on these lowground areas and the ffridd can also be reduced by housing a significant proportion of the ewes at lambing. Cattle also play an important role in the system, particularly through integrated grazing.

Resource management in hill flocks is undergoing great change since the introduction of the revised Common Agricultural Policy and the direction of UK Government support has shifted to environmental issues. Planning principles will become of greater importance as new opportunities for income become available and stock have to be managed with natural vegetation and wildlife in the newly created environmentally sensitive areas (ESA).

Table 8.9 Example of management plan to exploit resources. (Source: MAFF, 1981a)

	Ffridd and fields (130 ha of ffridd and 40 ha of fields)	Improved mountain (area 276 ha with 121 ha improved)	Unimproved mountain (area 210 ha)
January February March	Wintering of two year old ewes, weak ewes and crossbred ewes.	Wintering of ewes.	Wintering of ewes.
April	All ewes at lambing (proportion housed).	Rested and fertilized.	Grazing for yearlings on return from tack.
May June July	Grazing for ewes rearing crossbred twin lambs.	Grazing for ewes and lambs from mid April.	Grazing for yearlings and ewes not rearing rams.
August September	Grazing for ewe lambs from weaning until going to tack in early October. Fattening of wether lambs.	Grazing for two year old ewes.	Weaned ewes.
October November December	Flushing and tupping of ewes. Fattening of wether lambs.	Flushing and tupping ewes.	Rested.

9　Upland Sheep Production

The upland sheep flocks of Britain can be regarded as occupying an intermediate position between the extensive hill-grazed flocks and the large crossbred flocks of the lowland farms. This intermediate position not only refers to the part that the uplands play in the breeding structure of the British sheep industry but also to the physical characteristics of upland farms. The altitude of these farms, rainfall, soil type and pasture quality are all generally more suitable for sheep production than conditions found in hill areas, but nevertheless production potential can still be limited to some degree. While the physical attributes of upland farms occupy a position between those of hill and lowland areas, in reality there are no definite boundaries between them. The boundaries adopted in this chapter are those of the Hill Livestock Compensatory Allowance Scheme outlined in the introduction to Section 3.

Upland flocks contain about 17% of the United Kingdom breeding ewe population but play an important role in the national structure by supplying lowland farms with crossbred ewes. A large proportion of ewes in upland flocks are draft ewes from the hill areas. Over half of these are mated to Longwool rams such as the Border Leicester, Bluefaced Leicester or Teeswater to produce crossbred ewe lambs for sale to the lowlands. Crosses such as the North of England Mule, Scottish Mule, Masham, Scottish Halfbred, Welsh Mule and Greyface are some of the commonest found. Just under half of the draft hill ewes on upland farms are mated to Down rams, e.g. Suffolk, in order to produce lambs for slaughter. The remaining small proportion of draft hill ewes are mated with upland rams.

In general terms upland flocks are more productive than those in the hill areas, usually having higher levels of fertility and profitability. Hill ewes moved from hill grazings after their third or fourth crop receive a nutritional boost when moved to upland pastures, and produce more lambs. This is illustrated in Table 9.1 with data from

Table 9.1 Average performance of Scottish Blackface and Welsh Mountain ewes under hill and upland conditions. (Source: Weiner, 1979)

	Hill environment			Grassland farm		
	Weight (kg)	Fleece weight (kg)	Lambs reared per 100 ewes	Weight (kg)	Fleece weight (kg)	Lambs reared per 100 ewes
Scottish Blackface	41	1.7	81	67	2.6	151
Welsh Mountain	34	1.1	105	47	1.8	136

Weiner (1979). Hill ewes of the Scottish Blackface and Welsh Mountain breeds were compared on a grassland farm and the results are compared with those found from the same breeds under natural hill conditions. All aspects of performance, liveweight, fleece weight and rearing percentages were considerably better for both breeds under the more favourable upland conditions. A further illustration of this response to nutritional status is available from a trial at Redesdale EHF (Table 9.2). A hill flock, excluding two year old ewes, was divided at random into three groups; one third were left on the hill grazing, one third were moved to an enclosed hill area and offered self-feed blocks, and the final group were moved to reseeded pastures. After the first season, lamb production from the better pasture was

Table 9.2 Nutritional effects on lambing performance. (Source: MAFF, 1983)

	Grazing treatment		
	Hill grazing	Enclosed hill + feed blocks	Reseeded pasture
Per 100 ewes mated			
Empty ewes	6	6	2
Twin bearing ewes	16	32	51
Lambs born live and dead	109	126	149

considerably improved – an increase of 40%, due mainly to an increased number of twins but also to a lower incidence of barrenness. Condition scores and liveweights taken showed that while the ewes on the hill grazings were losing condition in the critical period prior to ram turn out, those on the reseeds maintained condition and therefore were more able to sustain increased ovulation rate and implantation.

Upland producers purchasing draft ewes from hill flocks and producing crossbed lambs to sell on as breeding females have exploited this nutritional response for many years. However, although this is the system of production most commonly associated with upland areas it is not the only one found in this type of environment. Further evidence of the levels of performance achieved from purebred ewes in upland flocks has already been shown in Table 4.2 with data from MLC's commercial flock records.

Products

Lambs are the major product from the upland flocks but their quality and number vary tremendously. Wool and some draft ewes may also contribute to the gross output of the flocks but they are a negligible component in the context of overall production. Flocks in upland areas also receive support grants in the form of ewe subsidies under the Less Favoured Area Directive, but this is paid at a lower rate than that applicable to the hill flocks. The relative contribution to gross output of the main factors in MLC recorded upland flocks selling finished and store lambs in 1991 is illustrated in Fig. 9.1. The results from flocks selling breeding ewe lambs are not included in the figures because the average price per breeding ewe lamb is significantly higher than that received for the slaughter or store lamb. This product of upland flocks, the breeding ewe lamb, merits consideration in more detail as it is a fundamental part of the lowland sheep sector of the industry.

The main components of the breeding structure in Britain have been outlined in Chapter 7. Approximately 10% of the total ewe population is involved in the production of crossbred females, involving the mating of an estimated 1.83 million draft hill ewes to longwool rams (see Fig. 7.2). The product of this sector of the industry is important both to the flocks undertaking its production and to the lowland producers making use of it in their own flock replacement plans. However, to the outside observer the various combinations between

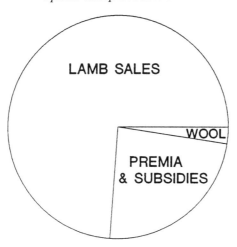

Fig. 9.1 Factors contributing to gross output in recorded upland flocks producing lambs from grass and forage in 1991. (Source: MLC, 1992a)

hill ewe and longwool ram create many crosses which at first may be confusing. They are produced as part of a deliberate flock policy which entails careful consideration of the potential markets and likely returns. The genetic background to the more important crossbreds is presented in Table 9.3. These are by no means the only examples, but in numerical terms they have the biggest influence on lowland sheep production.

Table 9.3 Examples of the more important crossbreds produced in upland flocks

Longwool ram	Hill ewe	Common name of female progeny	Main area of product
Border Leicester	Welsh Mountain	Welsh Halfbred	Wales
	Scottish Blackface	Greyface	Scotland
	North Country Cheviot	Scotch Halfbred	Scotland
	Hill Cheviot	Scotch Halfbred	Scotland
Bluefaced Leicester	Swaledale	North of England Mule	Northern England
	Scottish Blackface	North of England Mule	Northern England
	Scottish Blackface	Scottish Mule	Scotland
	Welsh Mountain	Welsh Mule	Wales
	Beulah	Welsh Mule	Wales
Teeswater	Swaledale	Masham	Northern England
	Dalesbred	Masham	Northern England

Some crossbred ewes have declined in popularity in recent years. A notable example is the Border Leicester × North Country Cheviot (Scotch Halfbred) ewe which in recent years has been replaced by Bluefaced Leicester crosses out of Swaledale and Scottish Blackface hill ewes. In a comparison of crossbred ewes from three longwool crossing sire breeds (Cameron, Smith & Deeble, 1983) a 6% litter size advantage of Bluefaced Leicester cross ewes over contemporary Border Leicester cross ewes was demonstrated. However, marketing factors such as more favourable breeding ewe prices and easier availability at a time when the ewe population was expanding are more probable reasons for the increased popularity of the Mule.

The Bluefaced Leicester breed has replaced the Border Leicester as the dominant Longwool crossing ram as a result of an increasing demand for cross rams. Interest in the breed and its crosses was centred in northern England until the early 1980s but the increasing supply of rams, coupled with a strong expansion of hill ewe numbers in Wales, has generated considerable interest in Bluefaced Leicester crosses out of the hardy Welsh breeds.

In the past eight to ten years a number of French breeds, such as the Rouge de l'Ouest and Bleu de Maine, have been imported to use as alternatives to the Bluefaced Leicester. Interest centred on their good conformation and carcase characteristics but the interest in their role as a sire of halfbred ewes has not increased significantly to challenge the place of the Bluefaced Leicester.

Production systems

It is extremly difficult to categorize sheep production in upland areas into particular systems. Results from MLC recorded flocks have shown that producers in these areas can achieve similar levels of profitability to lowland producers, and in fact the components of production which affect profitability in flocks selling finished and store lambs are similar to those which will be discussed for comparable lowland production systems in the next chapter (Table 9.4). However, the absolute levels of physical and financial performance differ between the two sectors, mainly because of the levels of nutrition and the higher level of flock inputs in the lowland sector. A comparison of performance figures for upland and lowland flocks selling similar products highlights the lower inputs made available to the upland flocks and the lower output which is obtained (Table 9.5).

Table 9.4 Contribution to top third superiority in gross margins per hectare for upland flocks selling finished and store lambs, 1991. (Source: MLC, 1992a)

	% contribution
Stocking rate	77
Number of lambs reared	8
Lamb sale price per head	3
Flock replacement costs	12

Table 9.5 Comparison of average performance characteristics of flocks selling finished and store lambs in uplands and lowlands. (Source: MLC, 1992a)

	Upland	Lowland
Lambs reared/ewe	1.37	1.52
Permanent pasture (%)	68.50	51.40
Grazing season (days)	181	192
Nitrogen use (kg/ewe)	8	10
Livestock unit grazing days/ha	370	518
Summer stocking rate (ewes/ha)	10.20	13.50
Concentrates (kg/ewe)	46	63
Lamb concentrates (kg/ewe)	5	14

A financial comparison suggests that there is little to choose between the two flock types in terms of overall profitability, measured by the gross margin per hectare (Table 9.6). Thus a low input/low output system is quite capable of producing similar returns to the alternative high input/high output type of system found in lowland areas. Of course, in the final analysis the former is probably more profitable because of the lower requirements in terms of working and fixed capital.

Flocks producing finished and store lambs
Reference has already been made to the diverse production systems in the uplands. Physical and financial results from MLC recorded flocks illustrate the average performance achieved and results from top third flocks point to possibilities for improvement (Table 9.7). The com-

Table 9.6 Comparison of average financial results of flocks selling finished and store lambs in upland and lowlands, 1991. (Source: MLC, 1992a)

	Upland (£/ewe)	Lowland (£/ewe)
Output	55.09	55.40
Costs:		
ewe and lamb concentrates	6.32	9.15
grassland costs	5.15	6.06
total feed and forage costs	11.63	15.84
Total variable costs	17.31	22.65
Gross margin	37.78	32.75
Gross margin per hectare (£)	389	432

ponents of profitability in these flocks for 1991 have been pointed out in Table 9.4. Top third flocks achieve increased output through higher lamb sales per ewe (a combination of more lambs reared per ewe and a higher lamb value) and a lower flock replacement cost. Top third flocks are therefore able to achieve considerably higher gross margins per hectare as a result of higher gross margins per ewe and higher stocking rates. The following example is provided to illustrate the type

Table 9.7 Average and top third results from upland flocks selling finished and store lambs, 1991. (Source: MLC, 1992a)

	Average	Top third
Physical		
Number of lambs reared per 100 ewes mated	137	140
Nitrogen use per hectare (kg)	80	101
Overall stocking rate (ewes/ha)	10.30	14.30
Nitrogen use per ewe (kg)	8	7
Financial		
Lamb sales (£/ewe)	44.40	46.60
Flock replacement cost (£/ewe)	7.58	5.15
Feed and forage costs (£/ewe)	11.63	11.73
Gross margin per ewe (£)	37.78	42.16
Gross margin per hectare (£)	389	603

of management involved and give some idea of the key components of production.

Example:

Beulah flock selling finished lambs off upland permanent pasture in conjunction with a small area of enclosed hill

---

Ewes are mated to Suffolk rams, apart from a small number mated pure for ewe replacements. Lambing is in March. Ewes are inwintered for approximately ten weeks and fed hay and silage. Lambs are sold off grass between June and November. The performance of the flock is presented in Table 9.8 together with target performance figures appropriate to this breed and system.

The flock has achieved a gross margin per hectare higher than target mainly as a result of significantly lower costs and despite a slightly lower number of lambs produced per ewe.

Performance figures presented in this way and compared with

Table 9.8 Specimen results for upland flocks selling finished and store lambs.

	Example Beulah flock	Target
Physical performance (per 100 ewes to ram)		
Number of empty ewes	4	4
Number lambs born alive	126	142
Number lambs reared	124	137
Summer stocking rate (ewes/ha)	14.4	10
Overall stocking rate (ewes/ha)	14	11
Financial performance (£/ewe)		
Lamb sales	42.9	41.0
Wool	1.6	1.6
Gross receipts	61.2	59.3
Less flock replacement cost	8.2	7.6
Gross output	53.0	51.7
Ewe and lamb concentrate costs	5.4	6.1
Fertilizer and forage costs	4.5	4.9
Total variable costs	15	17.3
Gross margin/ewe	38	34.4
Gross margin/ha	532	378

appropriate targets can identify the strengths and weaknesses of individual flocks. An examination of the reasons for a lower lamb crop may well reveal some aspect of ewe condition prior to tupping or ewe nutrition which could be improved in the future.

Flocks producing breeding ewe lambs

As discussed earlier, the number of flocks involved in the production of breeding females is a significant proportion of those found in the uplands. Many flocks of draft hill ewes could be mated to terminal sires to produce slaughter lambs, but there is an element of opportunism amongst producers and some opt to use longwool sires instead of conventional terminal sires because this gives them the chance to market crossbred ewe lambs for further breeding when conditions are favourable. This is the case in Scotland where considerably more Scottish Blackface ewes are mated to Border Leicester rams than is indicated by the number of Greyface ewe lambs coming on to the market. The practice is somewhat different in Wales where Suffolk cross Welsh or Beulah ewe lambs are sold as breeding replacements directly to the lowlands.

Results from MLC recorded flocks highlight the important differences between flocks selling breeding stock and those selling only finished and store lambs (Table 9.9). The marketing of breeding ewe lambs is a skilled operation. Lambs must be drawn and offered for sale in lots of equal type and size. The rewards from selling advantageously can be considerable; for example, in 1991 the total lamb sales per ewe for those flocks selling crossbred breeding stock ranged from £30 to £65 per ewe. The majority are sold through live auction markets local to the area of production, with prospective buyers travelling to these specialist breeding ewe sales from considerable distances. In many cases intermediaries are involved, buying on behalf of third parties or large breeder groups.

An inherent weakness of the crossbreeding system is the potential hazard from disease, particularly reproductive disorders such as abortion. There is an increasing trend for many crossbred lambs to be sold off breeders' farms, thus avoiding the central marketing system. This demands greater attention from the producer as potential customers wish to purchase from flocks with sound health records and a known veterinary history.

The following example illustrates the type of management involved and gives some idea of the key components of production.

Table 9.9 A comparison of two upland production systems in 1991. (Source: MLC, 1992a)

	Flocks selling slaughter/ store lambs	Flocks selling breeding stock
Financial results (£ per ewe)		
Gross receipts	63.08	61.88
Ewe replacement cost	7.53	7.80
Net output	55.55	54.08
Total feed and forage costs	12.00	10.40
Gross margin	37.67	38.64
Physical results (per 100 ewes)		
Lambs reared	139	130
Lambs sold or retained for:		
Slaughter	82	41
Breeding	12	41
Feeding	45	48

Example:

Swaledale flock run on leys and permanent pasture with access to a large area of enclosed hill ground

The main grazing season is short, commencing in early May and extending to the middle of October. Ewes are mated in early November to Bluefaced Leicester rams and one Swaledale ram solely for the production of flock replacements. Ewes are outwintered on sacrifice leys which are ploughed out in the spring.

Regrowths after silage cuts for the cattle enterprise are grazed by weaned lambs from August onwards. Crossbred lambs are sold in early September at a local breeding ewe sale and the remaining lambs, mainly castrates and small ewe lambs, are finished off the farm from weaning onwards.

Physical and financial performance figures are given for the flock in Table 9.10, along with target figures representing the average levels of performance achieved in flocks with a similar type of ewe and producing a similar type of product. Physical performance for the example flock was above average target levels with the result that a greater number of lambs were available for sale. However, stocking

Table 9.10 Specimen results for upland flocks selling breeding stock.

	Example Swaledale flock	Target
Physical performance (per 100 ewes to ram)		
Number of empty ewes	3	4
Number of lambs born alive	169	155
Number lambs reared	153	145
Summer stocking rate (ewes/ha)	9.5	10.0
Overall stocking rate (ewes/ha)	8.3	9.4
Financial performance (£/ewe)		
Lamb sales	49.0	45.2
Wool	1.6	1.5
Gross receipts	67.3	63.4
Less flock replacement cost	8.2	7.8
Gross output	59.1	55.6
Ewe and lamb concentrates	7.0	6.1
Fertilizer and forage costs	5.5	4.9
Total variable costs	17.2	16.0
Gross margin/ewe	41.9	39.6
Gross margin/ha	348	356

rates were below target levels. The overall financial results were lower than target despite a significantly higher gross margin per ewe. On examining the grassland production statistics, the low stocking rates can be accounted for by a lower than average nitrogen usage, i.e. 52 kg N/ha compared with an anticipated 80 kg N/ha.

10 Lowland Sheep Production

The lowland sector of the British sheep industry contributes the greatest proportion of finished lambs to the total output. This is a result of various production characteristics of the ewes involved and the better physical conditions found in the lowlands. An attempt has been made to highlight these strata differences in Table 10.1 where estimates of lamb carcase production are presented. Ewes in the lowland areas accounted for 48% of the breeding population in 1991 but, as a result of the relatively high output of finished lambs sold per ewe coupled with high average carcase weights, the proportion of total lamb carcase meat produced in this sector is estimated to be around 71%. The income derived from the end-products of the lowland ewe population generates much of the cash which filters through the industry to the hill and upland sectors.

It has been pointed out in Chapter 7 that the population in lowland areas consists to a large extent of crossbred ewes born in the upland regions. The regular buying of replacement breeding females from the uplands is an important link between the two sectors and a major

Table 10.1 Relative output from hill, upland and lowland sectors in Great Britain

	Breeding ewes 1991 (000 head)		Finished lambs sold/ewe	Average carcase weight (kg)	Total carcase weight (000 t)	
Hill	6692	(35%)	0.45	15	45	(12%)
Upland	3179	(17%)	1.1	18	63	(17%)
Lowland	9251	(48%)	1.5	19	264	(71%)
Total	19122				372	

source of funds for sheep producers in the uplands. Over 85% of lowland ewes originate in upland areas, 10% as purebred upland ewes and 75% as longwool crosses. The remaining 15% of lowland ewes are either purebred lowland ewes (13%) or terminal sire cross upland ewes. The financial interdependence between the lowland and upland sectors is seen elsewhere with the transfer of large volumes of store lambs, mainly wethers, from hill and upland farms to lowland units where they are finished on a whole range of different feed resources. These two large sources of animals from the hill and upland areas provide lowland sheep producers with considerable choice, particularly when the wide variety of origins and breeds are considered. This in turn gives the lowland producer scope for determining the type of lamb he wants to sell and a much greater opportunity to change his system of production. It is not surprising, therefore, that there is no one favoured system of production in lowland areas. Recorded data from the more popular systems highlights an enormous within system variation. Performance records from these systems of production provide invaluable advisory material for demonstrating the components of production which influence profitability.

Products

Gross output from lowland flocks is mainly derived from the sale of finished and store lambs, with a small contribution from wool. A number of flocks exist specifically to sell breeding stock, either rams or in some cases breeding females, but these are very much a minority in overall industry terms. Flockplan results from lowland spring lambing flocks selling lambs from grass in summer and autumn in 1991 illustrate the relative contribution of the main products to gross output (Fig. 10.1). The output of cull ewes from the flock merits some attention since an important outlay in British flocks is the flock replacement cost, components of which are the purchase price for replacement ewes, the level of ewe mortality, the average flock life and the price received for the cull ewe at the end of her productive life.

Finished lambs
Returns from finished lambs can significantly enhance overall gross margins if attention is paid to the factors which influence lamb returns, particularly marketing skills and the production of a more acceptable carcase. Requirements of both the UK home market and

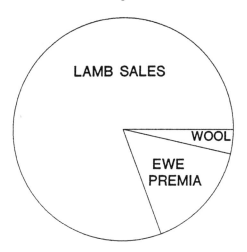

Fig. 10.1 Factors contributing to gross output in lowland flocks in 1991. (Source: MLC, 1992a)

export markets have become more precise and producers need to adapt their production to meet these market requirements, which are defined primarily in terms of lamb carcase weight and level of fat cover, more closely.

Weight requirements show quite wide variations. In Britain the main weight range is approximately 16–22 kg, with heavier carcases normally incurring a price penalty. The main European markets (Belgium, France and Germany) and the major British multiples require carcases in the narrower 16–19 kg range. In contrast, the Spanish and Italian markets prefer light lambs in the 8–12 kg weight range. By exploitation of the known variation in body size between different terminal sire breeds and the main ewe breeds and crossbreds, and the careful selection of lambs for slaughter, it is possible to increase the proportion of lambs falling into the required weight range.

Meat trade requirements for fatness levels are more uniform and are essentially for MLC fat classes 2 and 3L. Producers should therefore aim to produce as many lambs as possible within this target area for fatness while providing their particular outlet with the weight range of carcase required. Producers must be aware of particular market requirements and plan their production systems accordingly.

Store lambs for further fattening
It is common for many farm animals to be produced at one location and sold to a specialist finisher who will take them through to

slaughter. The sheep industry in Britain is no exception to this pattern, with around a quarter of the annual lamb crop being sold for further feeding on another farm. A major source of store lambs are hill flocks which have no resources for lamb finishing themselves. The production of store lambs can be a deliberate and viable enterprise plan in some lowland flocks and there are also lowland farms where slaughter lamb production is the main objective but where access to a store market acts as a useful safety valve if for any reason the main objective cannot be met. There are other flocks whose aim is to sell finished lambs and who fail in this objective.

Store lambs are available from any breed or cross and for the prospective purchaser represent an opportunity for profit. The lambs presented for sale by the producer must be such that the buyer can expect some scope for further fattening at a profit. Achieving a good price for store lambs involves careful selection and presentation. Batches have to be of even size and type to offer the potential customer an attractive financial proposition.

Wool

The importance of wool to the lowland producer has declined so much in recent years that wool sales now only represent 3% of the gross output from lowland flocks, compared to 8% in the early 1970s. In many situations returns are only enough to cover the expense of shearing. The British Wool Marketing Board is, of course, concerned that the national wool clip is harvested in good order so that the clip can be sold on the world markets. Care is still required when handling and managing ewes to ensure that as saleable a product as possible is produced. However, there is little scope for increasing flock output through improvement efforts directed at wool.

Cull ewes

The sale of ewes unsuitable for continued production is not a major source of income to the lowland flockmaster but returns can be improved with care and planning. Over 1.8 million cull ewes were slaughtered in 1982, yet until recently little was known about the reasons for culling or the methods of sale which were being adopted. A survey of Flockplan records produced some answers to these questions. Ewes were culled for a whole range of reasons with barrenness, accounting for 34% of batches, being the most common. A wide range of age related factors, including loss of teeth, poor udders and general poor body condition, accounted for the remainder.

Table 10.2 The seasonal pattern of cull ewe sales and prices, 1981–2. (Source: MLC, 1983)

	% of batches	% of all ewe sales	Av. batch size	Av. price per ewe (£)
December 1981	1.1	0.2	3	16.68
January 1982	3.8	1.8	7	28.83
February	5.8	2	5	26.26
March	12.1	6	7	27.36
April	20	14	10	26.51
May	10.3	6.6	9	24.32
June	7.4	5.4	10	19.51
July	8.2	8.4	15	18.97
August	9.9	14.2	21	18.97
September	9.5	24.2	36	21.24
October	8.1	10.1	18	19.83
November	3.8	7.2	27	20.09

The survey revealed an important variation in cull ewe prices (Table 10.2). These did not follow the pattern of cull ewe sales but reflected the seasonal lamb price pattern, the highest prices being paid early in the year and the lowest in July and August.

Returns for cull ewes can, therefore, be improved if they are sold as early in the year as possible. Pregnancy diagnosis, which was referred to earlier, is valuable in the identification of barren ewes at an early stage. Where ewes are culled in the autumn some consideration should be given to maintaining them in good condition over the winter to sell when prices are at a peak. It also appeared from the survey that ewes presented for sale in even size lots received higher prices.

The destination of cull ewes once they have left the farm becomes speculative. A strong trade for ewes exists between Britain and France, with both carcases and live ewes being shipped over in some numbers. On the domestic market there is a strong demand from Asian communities, particularly in the Midlands and south-eastern conurbations of England.

Breeding stock

Two important purebred groups are found in the lowland sector: those producing terminal sires for use on crossbred ewe flocks, and those producing breeding females for sale as either ewe lambs or two year olds. The former group of terminal sire breeds, of which the Suffolk is a notable example, are scattered throughout Britain and make somewhere in excess of 40 000 young crossing rams a year available to the industry. The majority of such flocks rely on ram sales as their major source of income, but unfortunately the type of financial data available from the Flockplan scheme for commercial flocks is not available for these ram producing flocks.

The purebred flocks producing breeding females of various ages are also difficult to describe in financial terms. They are generally localized breeds, and some have characteristics of particular interest. The Dorset Horn and Poll Dorset ewe, for example, are popular in the south-west of England and are notable for their extended breeding season. Large flocks lambing from 60–80% of the ewes in October and November and the remainder in the early spring produce a significant number of young milk-fed lambs which are marketed at Easter.

The Lleyn breed, from the peninsula of that name in North Wales, is another lowland breed which has risen in popularity as a commercial lowland ewe at a phenomenal rate since the early 1970s when it was considered as a potential rare breed by the Rare Breed Survival Trust. The characteristics which have brought it to its present heights of popularity are low mature size, high prolificacy and precocity in the ewe lambs, which when combined are desirable characteristics for commercial ewes.

Production systems

The aim of the sheep farmer in the lowlands is to combine the various elements of the production system in order to sell lambs at a price greater than their cost of production. His achievements are as variable as the systems available to him. Three factors are of crucial importance on lowland sheep systems: the feed resources available for the flock, the characteristics of the product that the producer aims to market and his expected returns from the market for that product.

The importance of grassland to sheep production has already been discussed. The main grazing season extends from about late March to early October in most areas and, as has been highlighted, the grass has the most nutritional value in this period. It can also be used as a source of food during the winter months either as a conserved product or as a standing crop. As it is the cheapest and most convenient source of nutrition, the objective of most lowland systems is to make the best strategic use of grass throughout the year. However, there are other sources of grazing available which include stubbles, early bite of winter cereals, catch crops and root crops. These are usually used to augment the feed available from grass and in many cases fit into an overall farming pattern which utilizes resources that would otherwise be wasted. The overall objective is for the producer to maximize his returns from the whole farm.

The main types of product that can be produced in the lowland flock have been outlined earlier in this chapter. However, such a variety of products means that production must be carefully planned in order to achieve the required output. There may not be much difference between a fat class 4 and a fat class 5 lamb but the financial penalties for producing the latter are heavy. Thus it is important to define the product that is to be produced and devise the best system possible to produce this product.

Since the removal of the sheep variable premium scheme in January 1992 returns for slaughter lambs have not been as predictable. However, the representative price for the main liveweight bands of lambs sold at auction, referred to as the standard quality quotation (SQQ) followed a broadly similar trend to market prices in previous years (Table 10.3). The variability of lamb price throughout the year offers scope for adapting production systems to achieve the best returns from a flock.

It needs to be said from the outset that the four lowland systems of production outlined here are generalizations towards which the majority of lowland flocks tend to conform. They are perhaps the ideal but each producer has his own way of improving some aspect of

Table 10.3 Average market prices in Great Britain, 1992–3

Month	SQQ (p/kg/weight)	Month	SQQ (p/kg/weight)
April	95.1	October	74.6
May	80.0	November	73.7
June	87.9	December	80.5
July	76.4	January	90.1
August	74.0	February	111.0
September	71.4	March	126.0

SQQ: Standard quality quotation

them. Certain elements of all the systems are part of a continuum. It can be dangerous or misleading to talk of early lambing and spring lambing flocks, for example, as if they have completely separate characteristics when in reality lambing dates are spread from October through to April with major clusters at certain times. Similarly flocks who in retrospect may best be described as store lamb producing flocks may in fact be slaughter lamb producers whose production plans have failed. As was mentioned in Chapter 1, there are no blueprints for success. The following are offered only as examples of certain recognizable production systems.

Early lambing systems

The primary objective of the early lamb producer is to market lambs at a time when prices are highest. This involves mating ewes in August and early September to lamb in January, and selling lambs from March onwards. Ewes are weaned early and therefore it is possible to stock ewes more heavily during the grazing season. Other advantages include the better utilization of skilled labour at a time of year when it may otherwise be underutilized. Buildings may be used for longer periods than would otherwise be the case and the contribution of the sheep enterprise to the overall farm cash flow profile may be greater.

However, there are also some difficulties to be overcome. The ovulation rate of sheep mated this early in the season is likely to be lower and the greater dependency on housing increases feed requirements. It is therefore a high input/high output system, with obvious dangers if anticipated returns are not achieved. A similar argument holds for the indoor-fed lambs. There may be a greater disease risk because of the intense system of management and therefore a higher level of management and supervision is required.

Despite these difficulties, early lambing can be a viable proposition provided that attention is paid to these critical areas. The factors which contribute to profitability in early flocks recorded by MLC in 1991 are illustrated in Table 10.4 which shows the contribution to top third superiority in gross margin per hectare.

The number of lambs reared, lamb sale price per head and stocking rate were the most important aspects of early lamb production. Lamb rearing in early lambing flocks involves either early weaning and housing to slaughter on a high quality concentrate diet, or alternatively finishing on grass with high levels of concentrate feeding to help early growth. This second method of lamb finishing is more appropriate for flocks lambing in January and early February. Both systems depend on high concentrate usage to maximize growth to

Table 10.4 Percentage contribution to top third superiority in gross margin per hectare for early lambing flocks, 1991. (Source: MLC, 1992a)

	% contribution
Lamb sale price per head	7
Number of lambs reared	15
Feed and forage costs	15
Stocking rate	59
Other factors	4

slaughter. Top third flocks had, in fact, higher feed and forage costs than average. Performance levels for flocks which early wean lambs and finish them indoors and those finishing lambs at grass are presented in Table 10.5. Figures for average lowland grass finishing flocks are presented alongside for comparison.

Table 10.5 Comparison of results from two early lambing and lowland grass finished systems. (Source: MLC, 1992a)

	Early lambing		Lowland grass finished
	Lambs fed indoors on concentrates	Lambs reared on grass	
Financial results			
Lamb sales/ewe (£)	66.50	60.20	50.60
Lamb feed costs/ewe (£)	16.40	8.30	1.60
Gross margin/ewe (£)	34.30	36.50	32.80
Gross margin/ha (£)	596	536	432
Physical results			
Lambs reared/ewe	1.50	1.44	1.52
Stocking rate (ewe/ha)	17.40	14.70	13.20
Kg nitrogen/ewe	7	9	10
Percentage of lambs sold			
Feb. and March	35	20	0
April and May	52	35	3
June and July	13	31	24
July and Aug.	0	10	23
Sept. and Oct.	0	2	8

Early lamb production systems can be more profitable on a per hectare basis than the more conventional March and April lambing systems provided that the high levels of lamb concentrate usage lead to early lamb sales in April and May when sale value per lamb is at its highest.

Breed choice is important to the success of these systems. Certain breeds of ewe, such as the Dorset Horn, have the ability to conceive at most times of the year and they are used in some cases. The Finnish Landrace crossed onto the Dorset Horn or Poll Dorset is an alternative which combines the extensive breeding season of the Dorset with the higher prolificacy of the Finnish Landrace. Ewes out of any of the common crossbreds sired by Suffolk rams are also popular, mainly because of their earlier breeding season but also for their excellent conformation. Rams of the medium size ram breeds such as the Charollais are the most popular choice of sire because they reach their optimum weight and level of carcase finish earlier than some of the larger terminal sire breeds. Quality lambs can then be marketed in April, May and June.

Example:
January lambing Finnish Landrace × Dorset Horn ewes mated to Charollais rams. The lambs are early weaned and fed on concentrates for an early sale.

Although the flock reared slightly more lambs than the target figures (Table 10.6), crossbred ewes of this type ought to be able to rear 160%. The financial return from lamb sales was better than the target, indicating that one of the main objectives of this system, i.e. selling lambs on the high-priced Easter lamb market, was achieved. This target selling pattern was achieved at a price, as is shown by the high level of concentrates used by the ewes and lambs. Lamb concentrate costs in early weaning systems where the lambs are fed indoors should not be affected by the different climatic conditions found in different years. Ewes, however, will react much more to the prevailing climate, and when autumn grazing is poor and the winter harsh, early lambing systems rely heavily on ewe concentrates to keep ewes in condition for lambing and lactation.

The example flock also managed to achieve one of the other objectives of this system: high stocking rates at grass during the summer grazing season. This incurred a slightly higher fertilizer and

Table 10.6 Specimen results for early lambing flocks finishing lambs on concentrates

	Example Finn × Dorset flock	Target
Physical performance (per 100 ewes to ram)		
Number of empty ewes	4	5
Number of lambs born alive	151	157
Number of lambs reared	148	150
Summer stocking rate (ewes/ha)	22.80	20.00
Overall stocking rate (ewes/ha)	21	18
Financial performance (£/ewe)		
Lamb sales	72.50	68.84
Wool	2.50	2.26
Ewe premium	10.50	10.47
Gross receipts	85.50	81.57
Less flock replacement cost	7.63	6.45
Gross output	77.87	75.12
Ewe and lamb concentrate costs	29.80	26.91
Fertilizer and forage costs	5.20	4.80
Total variable costs	46.00	40.28
Gross margin/ewe	31.87	34.84
Gross margin/ha	669	627

forage cost than the target figures. The gross margin per ewe was below target due to the high feed costs, but the gross margin per hectare was good as a result of the high level of grassland management achieved. This flock could probably make a better use of concentrate feeds and should be able to achieve a better lamb output from such a prolific type of ewe.

Spring lambing flocks

Lambs from grass

The production of finished lambs from grass in lowland flocks is just as much a response to physical conditions as are the production systems found in upland and hill areas. In the case of the lowland flocks, however, the physical determinants of the system are not so much climatic as biological. The use of early season grass as a source of high quality nutrients, both for the milking ewe and for the young growing lamb, as well as the declining quality of summer grazing each in their ways determine the system.

The key management factors are the correct feeding of the ewe throughout her life cycle, good grassland management and the ability to finish lambs quickly at acceptable market weights. As mentioned in Chapter 4, there are two key times in the ewe's life cycle towards which correct feeding is aimed: mating and birth. By developing a good pre-mating flushing technique it is possible to encourage the ewe to shed the optimum number of eggs and to implant them successfully in their fertilized state. Similarly the climax of nutrition is aimed at allowing the ewe to deliver a healthy pair of twins in such a condition that she can provide adequate milk to rear them and they are fit to take the full benefit of that milk supply. Good grassland management helps this process, not only by supplying the high quality grazing just after birth but also by providing a good quality winter feed in the form of hay or silage.

Records from lowland spring lambing flocks recording with MLC in 1991 highlight the important factors which influence profitability (Table 10.7). Stocking rate is the most important component of success and has been for a number of years, but this is not too surprising as stocking rate directly influences gross margin per hectare and this is the performance criterion used to select the top third flocks.

The recording of commercial enterprises in Britain has emphasized the wide variation in results achieved in practice and the close relationship between physical performance and gross margins. Stocking rates have been one of the main performance characters to show a consistent rise, demonstrating the producers' ability to improve their use of farm resources and exploit this variation.

Results from MLC recorded flocks in 1991 show that flocks in the top third category were able to spend more per hectare to grow the

Table 10.7 Percentage contribution to top third superiority in gross margin per hectare for lowland spring lambing flocks. (Source: MLC, 1992a)

	% contribution
Lamb sale price/head	3
Number of lambs reared	8
Flock replacement costs	12
Stocking rate	77

Table 10.8 Comparison of grassland costs, utilization and production of conserved forage in top third lowland spring lambing flocks (Average = 100). (Source: MLC, 1984a)

Variable costs of grass production (£/ha)	108
Percentage of grass production costs spent on fertilizer	103
Conserved forage yields (tonnes/ha)	
Hay	116
Silage	111
Grassland stocking rate (ewes/ha)	123
Grassland costs (£ per ewe)	87

grass and yet to exploit these additional feed resources and stock their ewes more intensively (Table 10.8). A comparison of grassland costs and production between average and top third flocks shows the cost of grass production in the more efficient flocks to be less per ewe than for average flocks, and the amount of nitrogen used per ewe is similar.

The average number of grazing days in MLC recorded lowland flocks is about 192, thus lambs finished at grass must reach the required market weight within this time span. The finishing period is a function of several factors which include date of birth, genotype and nutritional status or grassland availability,. The percentage of lambs sold in two-monthly periods in recorded flocks illustrates the typical marketing pattern found in these flocks (see Table 10.5).

Lambing dates are largely determined by the time that grass growth commences, enabling ewes and young lambs to be turned out to fresh young grass. In lowland Britain this means a March turn out date (60% of recorded flocks lamb in March) and fixes the possible growth period at between three and five months. The choice of terminal sire breed is important. Rams that will produce fast growing lambs to finish at between 16 and 18 kg are required. Breeds with an adult bodyweight of between 80 and 90 kg are suitable for this purpose, the Charollais being a good example. The larger Suffolk and Texel rams are widely used in this system but lambs will need to be finished at fat class 2 rather than fat class 3 if a large proportion are to be sold off grass. Whatever the breed chosen it is essential to buy rams with good performance records as a ram with a fast lean growth rate itself has the ability to pass this on to its offspring.

Irrespective of the lamb's genetic potential for growth, it is essential to remove all checks and constraints so that the lamb may attain that potential. Feeding is an important element. The importance of body condition prior to mating and ewe nutrition in the late stages of pregnancy and through the early phase of lactation have already been stressed and discussed in detail. Attention to these factors does not necessarily mean higher feed costs. Top third flocks use lower amounts of ewe concentrate, contributing less to the variable cost of production. This suggests that successful flockmasters have a greater awareness of the critical periods of nutrition and that they are able to control slightly lower feed resources more precisely. A comparison of the more important feed costs for average and top third flocks highlights these points (Table 10.9). Many producers overlook the importance of lamb creep in relation to the end price for the lamb.

Example:

Suffolk rams used on Scotch Halfbred ewes to lamb in mid-March. All lambs to be sold from grass during the summer at 18.5 kg carcase weight. Ewes fed on a catch crop in the autumn as part of an arable cropping system.

The key profitability factors in the example (Table 10.10) are the good grassland management demonstrated by the flock and the high return per lamb achieved. The lambing and rearing performance of this flock is disappointing considering the potential of the crossbred ewe involved; flocks of this type should rear 170%. The average lamb price achieved was £34.67 compared with the target of £33.93. This was made possible through a group marketing scheme which earns a premium for producers selling lambs to a very precise specification on

Table 10.9 Ewe and lamb concentrate costs in average and top third lowland flocks 1991. (Source: MLC, 1992a)

	Average	Top third
Concentrate usage per ewe (kg)	63	65
Average ewe concentrate cost (£/tonne)	120	110
Ewe concentrate cost (£/ewe)	7.53	7.10
Lamb concentrate usage (kg)	12	17
Average lamb concentrate cost (£/tonne)	135	116
Lamb concentrate cost (£/ewe)	1.62	1.98

Table 10.10 Specimen results for lowland flocks selling finished lambs from grass

	Example Scotch Halfbred flock	Target
Physical performance (per 100 ewes to ram)		
Number of empty ewes	3	5
Number of lambs born alive	154	157
Number of lambs reared	150	152
Summer stocking rate (ewes/ha)	20.10	16.00
Overall stocking rate (ewes/ha)	17.80	13.50
Financial performance (£/ewe)		
Lamb sales	52.00	51.85
Wool	2.30	2.25
Ewe premium	10.70	9.88
Gross receipts	65.00	63.98
Less flock replacement cost	6.30	7.40
Gross output	58.70	56.58
Ewe and lamb concentrate costs	18.00	10.15
Fertilizer and forage costs	2.10	5.78
Total variable costs	24.40	22.76
Gross margin/ewe	40.60	41.22
Gross margin/ha	723	556

a regular basis. In addition, the producer buys his Suffolk rams from a breeder with reliable performance data and thus can select rams with good performance characteristics. Concentrate costs were nearly double the target figures but the high lamb growth rates achieved to some extent justify this.

A high level of grassland management is shown by low fertilizer and forage costs per ewe generating a better-than-target stocking rate. This turned a moderately good gross margin per ewe into a very good result. The only weakness of this flock appears to be the rearing percentage of the ewes.

Lambs from grass and forage crops

The finishing of lambs from forage crops in late summer and autumn may be carried out for one of several reasons. Local market requirements may demand a heavier weight of lamb than can be produced from grass. The breeds of both ewes and rams may allow a heavier weight of lamb to be produced which will then compete for the grassland resources with the ewes. Grazing conditions may be such that an alternative source of good quality feed is required during the late summer or autumn. Whatever the reason for adopting this system to produce finished lambs, the essentials are the same. Good lamb growth achieved at grass should be maintained when lambs are transferred on to the forage crop which must be in plentiful supply. Finishing lambs from forage crops relies on the principles of lamb production previously discussed. These include good levels of production from grass (including optimal ewe nutrition), good grassland management and utilization and attention to the market weights to which the lambs are to be taken.

A range of crops are available for use in this system including stubble turnips, undersown cereals or late spring brassicas such as kale and rape. Some crops are more suited to particular farm situations than others and, provided that plans are made to ensure an adequate supply, any crop will do. On the other hand some crops are not cheap to grow, thus a careful matching of lamb requirements to the amount of feed provided is of paramount importance to ensure full and profitable utilization.

The production of lambs from forage crops is an alternative to finishing lambs from grass in most lowland situations but in many cases it is second best. Generally, the profitability of flocks producing lambs from forage crops is never as good as those producing lambs from grass. In some situations, however, farm circumstances or climatic conditions may mean that finishing lambs from forage crops is a more attractive proposition than grass finishing.

Of the system employed incorporating forage crops into the farm rotation in conjunction with grass, three different objectives can be recognized. There are those farms which utilize forage crops to finish lambs in the autumn; there are those which sell mainly store lambs from their system and, through forage crop utilization, reduce the number of lambs sold from the farm as stores; and there is a third category which actually retain their lambs for further finishing later in the year in a more specific lamb finishing system. The relative profitability of these different systems and the different lamb production patterns are shown in Table 10.11 along with results from flocks selling the majority of their lambs as finished lambs from grass.

Although flocks selling their lambs from grass and forage received a higher return for their lambs, the extra cost of growing the forage

Table 10.11 Lamb finishing systems in lowland spring lambing flocks 1989. (Source: MLC, 1990)

	Finished lamb flocks		Store lamb selling flocks	Store lamb finishing flocks
	Grass	Forage	Forage	Forage
Lamb sales per ewe (£)	56.31	59.81	51.90	55.21
Feed and forage costs per ewe (£)	15.10	17.09	17.96	15.24
Gross margin per ewe (£)	35.33	37.58	27.05	33.75
Gross margin per hectare (£)	482	411	299	414
Summer stocking rate (ewes/ha)	14.30	13.40	13.00	13.80
Overall stocking rate (ewes/ha)	14.20	11.20	10.70	12.20
Lambs per 100 ewes to ram				
Reared	143	149	150	144
Sold finished	102	113	52	61
Sold or retained for feeding	32	27	90	69

crops reduced this advantage. Grass and forage flocks also had lower overall stocking rates than grass only flocks, and thus their overall gross margin per hectare was some £71 less. Flocks selling store lambs from forage crops were a lot less profitable than those selling finished lambs due to lower lamb sales.

Example:

Greyface ewes mated to a larger type of Suffolk ram to lamb in early April. Lambs to be finished at 22 kg of carcase weight mainly from a root crop in the winter.

This example flock fell well below target in several key areas (Table 10.12) including rearing percentage, lamb sales and forage crop management. Profitability was maintained at a respectable level by good summer grazing management and a low level of variable costs.

Table 10.12 Specimen results for lowland flocks selling lambs from forage crops

	Example Greyface flock	Target
Physical performance (per 100 ewes to ram)		
Number of empty ewes	4	5
Number of lambs born alive	150	158
Number of lambs reared	142	152
Summer stocking rate (ewes/ha)	21.80	17.50
Overall stocking rate (ewes/ha)	14.90	12.30
Financial performance (£/ewe)		
Lamb sales	46.00	51.78
Wool	1.90	2.10
Ewe premium	9.80	10.10
Gross receipts	57.70	63.98
Less flock replacement cost	7.72	6.11
Gross output	49.98	57.87
Ewe and lamb concentrate costs	6.90	9.16
Fertilizer and forage costs	4.20	6.72
Total variable costs	16.80	22.83
Gross margin/ewe	33.20	35.04
Gross margin/ha	494	506

The poor rearing percentage contributed towards the poor lamb sales results, but the lambs did not achieve the prices expected of them either. A poor establishment of the swedes grown as part of the finishing diet, and thus a low stocking rate on the forage crop, meant that lambs had to be sold at a less than optimum weight. This is also reflected in the large difference between the summer stocking rate and overall stocking rate.

Ewe and lamb concentrate costs were low. In such a system little concentrate would be fed to the lambs and in this case a low level was fed to the ewes also. Gross margin per ewe was moderate and the gross margin per hectare was only saved from being poor by the good use of grass during the summer. This system is obviously more prone to poor growing conditions, and once in a difficult situation it is expensive to maintain flock performance.

Lamb finishing

Lambs sold through the autumn and winter periods finished on a wide variety of feed resources originate from all sectors of the sheep industry. A large proportion are purchased in the store lamb markets at the end of the main grazing period while others are finished on their farm of origin. The traditional store lamb can be any one of three basic types: purebred hill lambs from the hill areas, longwool cross lambs out of the hill ewes produced in the upland areas, and finally lambs out of the crossbred ewe population in the lowlands. The first two groups are predominantly wether or castrate lambs.

Producers intending to operate a lamb finishing enterprise and faced with these variable animal resources must forward plan carefully. The availability of suitable feed must match the animals' requirements if lambs are to be marketed economically and thus provide some return. MLC recorded lamb finishing enterprises highlight a number of the more important components of profitability (Table 10.13). Financial and physical performance factors presented for average and top third flocks in 1987–8 show the feeders margin to be the largest difference between the two groups. Top third flocks bought lambs for a little more but were able to achieve a higher end price through retaining lambs for on average two weeks longer to achieve the higher prices prevailing later in the season. While this delayed marketing increased returns, there are some dangers from

Table 10.13 Performance of store lamb finishing enterprises. (Source: MLC, 1988c)

	Average (£/lamb)	Top-third (£/lamb)
Output		
Lamb sales	44.80	48.71
Less lamb purchase price	33.45	35.14
Feeders margin	9.35	13.57
Total variable costs	3.34	3.21
Gross margin per lamb	6.01	10.36
Physical performance		
Average group size	671	610
Average number of days feeding	106	117
Feed cost/lamb/week (p)	18	15
Mortality (%)	2.0	1.3

producing lambs which are too fat for market demands and therefore a possibility that penalties may be incurred. Top third flocks also feed their lambs more economically – 3p less per lamb per week than average.

Feed resources made available to the enterprise will depend on the availability of grass and in the case of forage crops the soil type, climate and restrictions on crop rotation. Forward lambs (those close to their optimum slaughter weight) may use autumn grass and/or rape, while small hill lambs and the larger cross lambs out of the upland and lowlands are more ideally suited for sale from January onwards when the market prices can be expected to be higher. Specialist crops such as turnips, rape or swedes are therefore required or alternatively, if the relationships between concentrate and barley prices and lamb prices are favourable, the *ad lib* feeding of barley may be considered.

Variable costs of production of the crop influence profitability but with the wide variation of crop yields occurring in practice it is difficult to be precise on exact costs. Whatever the production costs, the potential of the standing crop has to be fully exploited and some guidance can be given in this area provided that the crop yield is available. It is therefore essential that square metre samples of the crop are weighed in order to give a reliable assessment. Recommended potential stocking rates according to yield, type of lamb, crop utilization and the supplementation of concentrates for rape and soft turnips (stubble and yellow fleshed varieties) have been discussed in Chapter 5.

As an alternative to finishing lambs on grass and forage crops, lambs can be finished indoors on silage based diets provided that the silage is well made. This type of finishing system is most appropriate for large hill and crossbred lambs with a potential to gain upwards of 15 kg after the supply of autumn grass is exhausted.

The late born and small types of hill lamb are probably more suited to an indoor finishing system. Growth rates of up to 200 gms per day are possible with the larger crossbred lambs while slightly lower gains with the smaller hill lambs are likely. This type of lamb finishing enterprise is entirely dependent on the price of concentrates in relation to the end price for the lamb. Results from MLC recorded units in 1983 illustrate the important physical and financial performance from four different systems of finishing (Table 10.14). The Suffolk cross lambs kept until late winter and finished on forage crops were the most profitable due to the combination of a good weight of lamb and

Table 10.14 Results for different store lamb types and systems, 1983–4. (Source: MLC, 1984b)

	Suffolk cross lambs sold off grass and forage in late autumn	Suffolk cross lambs sold off forage in winter	Housed lambs	Hill lambs
Financial (£/lamb)				
Lamb sales	38.09	45.08	38.60	38.66
Less lamb purchases	32.50	31.28	28.08	26.87
Feeders margin	5.59	13.80	10.52	11.79
Purchased feed	1.58	2.39	5.14	3.84
Grass costs	0.05	0.24	0.13	0.62
Forage crop costs	0.50	1.99		1.42
Total feed and forage	2.13	4.62	5.27	5.88
Total variable costs	2.40	5.44	5.74	6.89
Gross margin	3.19	8.36	4.78	4.90
Physical results				
Average no. of lambs	428	464	305	1433
Overall days	116	175	120	146
Average no. of days	57	129	74	124
Lamb mortality (%)	0.7	1.5	1.4	2.1
Concentrates/lamb (kg)	12	15	31	23
Feed cost/week (p)	32	20	81	17

high market prices. The short-keep Suffolk lambs had a low gross margin due to the narrow feeders margin while the housed and hill lambs had good feeders margins but higher feed costs.

References

Allen, P. (1990) New approaches to measuring body composition in live meat animals. In: *Reducing Fat in Meat Animals*. (eds J.D. Wood & A.V. Fisher). Elsevier Applied Science, London.

Armstrong, R.H., Eadie, J. & Maxwell, T.J. (1978) The development and assessment of a modified hill sheep production system at Sourhope, in the Cheviot Hills (1968–76). HFRO *7th Report 1974–76*. Hill Farming Research Organisation, Edinburgh.

ATB (1989) *Artificial Insemination of Sheep*. Agricultural Training Board, West Wickham.

Cameron, N.D., Smith, C. & Deeble, F.K. (1983) Comparative performance of crossbred ewes from three crossing sire breeds. *Animal Production*, **37**, 415–21.

Cockrem, F.R.M. (1979) A review of the influence of liveweight and flushing on fertility made in the context of efficient sheep production. *Proceedings of the New Zealand Society of Animal Production*, **39**, 23–42.

Corrall, A.J. (1983) *Efficient Grassland Farming*. British Grassland Society, Reading.

Croston, D., Danell, O., Elsen, J.M., Flamant, J.C., Hanrahan, J.P., Jakubec, V., Nitter, G. & Trodahl, S. (1980) A review of sheep recording and evaluation of breeding animals in European Countries: a group report. *Livestock Production Science*, **7**, 373–92.

Croston, D. & Guy, D.R. (1990) Review of the application of selection indices to meat sheep in Europe. *41st Annual Meeting of European Association for Animal Production, Toulouse*.

Croston, D., Kempster, A.J., Guy, D.R. & Jones, D.W. (1987) Carcass composition of crossbred lambs by ten sire breeds compared at the same carcass subcutaneous fat proportion. *Animal Production*, **44**, 99–106.

Croston, D. & Owen, M.G. (1992) Ultrasonic evaluation of live sheep in breeding programmes. *43rd Annual Meeting of European Association for Animal Production*, Madrid.

Cuthbertson, A. (1993) Technical developments in carcass classification, grading and identification systems. In: *Meat Strategies. The sheepmeat industry: structure and technology*. Meat and Livestock Commission, Milton Keynes.

Cuthbertson, A., Croston, D. & Jones, D.W. (1983) In vivo estimation of lamb carcass composition and lean tissue growth rate. In: *In Vivo Measurement of Body Composition in Meat Animals*. (ed. D. Lister). Elsevier Applied Science, London.

EDCA (1973) *Hills and Uplands, UK Farming and the Common Market*. Economic Development Committee for Agriculture, National Economic Development Office, UK.

FAO (1991) *1990 FAO Production Yearbook*, Vol. **44**, Food and Agriculture Organisation, Rome.

Fitzgerald, S. (1983) The use of forage crops for store lamb fattening. In: *Sheep Production*. (ed. W. Haresign) pp. 239–86. Butterworths, London.

Forbes, T.J., Dibb, C., Green, J.O., Hopkins, A. & Peel, S. (1980) *Factors Affecting the Productivity of Permanent Grassland*. Agricultural Development and Advisory Service/Grassland Research Institute, Maidenhead.

France, J., Neal, H.D., St.C. & Pollott, G.E. (1982) Using a programmable calculator for rationing pregnant ewes. *Agricultural Systems*, **9**, 267–79.

Grant, S.A. & King, J. (1984) Grazing management and pasture production: the importance of sward morphological adaptations and canopy photosynthesis. *HFRO Biennial Report 1982–3*. Hill Farming Research Organisation, Edinburgh.

Guy, D.R., Croston, D., Jones, D.W., Williams, G.L. & Cameron, N.D. (1986) Response to Selection in Welsh Mountain Sheep. *Animal Production*, **42**, 442 (abstract).

Hughes, R. (1976) Hills and uplands in Britain – The limitations and the development of potential. In: *Hill Lands Proc. of an International Symposium*. West Virginia University Books, Morgantown.

Ingram, J. (1990) The potential yield and varietal choice available for the major forage crops. In: Milk and Meat From Forage Crops, (ed. G.E. Pollott), *BGS Occasional Symposium No. 24*. British Grassland Society, Reading.

IWS (1983) *Wool Facts*. International Wool Secretariat, Bradford.

IWS (1992) *Wool Facts*. International Wool Secretariat, Bradford.

Kempster, A.J., Croston, D., Guy, D.R. & Jones, D.W. (1987) Growth and carcass characteristics of crossbred lambs by ten sire breeds, compared at the same estimated subcutaneous fat proportion. *Animal Production*, **44**, 83–98.

Kempster, A.J., Croston, D. & Jones, D.W. (1982) Value of conformation as an indicator of sheep carcass composition within and between breeds. *Animal Production*, **33**, 39–50.

Land, R.B., Atkins, K.D. & Roberts, R.C. (1983) Genetic improvement of reproductive performance. In: *Sheep Production*. (ed. W. Haresign), pp. 515–36. Butterworths, London.

Linklater, K.A. & Watson, G.A.L. (1983) Sheep housing and health. *The Veterinary Record*, **113**, 560–64.

Maxwell, T.J. & Treacher, T.T. (1987) Decision rules for grassland management. In: Efficient sheep production from grass, (ed. G.E. Pollott), *BGS Occasional Symposium No. 21*. British Grassland Society, Reading.

MAFF (1977) *The Changing Structure of Agriculture 1968–1975*. HMSO, London.

MAFF (1980) *Redesdale EHF Annual Review 1980*. HMSO, London.

MAFF (1981a) Systems for Welsh Mountain Sheep. *Booklet 2323*. Ministry of Agriculture, Food and Fisheries, Middlesex.

MAFF (1981b) *Redesdale EHF Annual Review 1981*. HMSO, London.

MAFF (1983) *Redesdale EHF Annual Review 1983*. HMSO, London.

Mills, Olivia (1989) *Practical Sheep Dairying*. Thorsons, Wellingborough.

MLC (1979) *Data Summaries on Upland and Lowland Sheep Production*. Meat & Livestock Commission, Milton Keynes.

MLC (1980a) *Retail Meat Cuts in Great Britain*. Meat & Livestock Commission, Milton Keynes.

MLC (1980b) *Commercial Sheep Production Yearbook. 1979–80*. Meat & Livestock Commission, Milton Keynes.

MLC (1982) *Sheep Artificial Insemination*. Meat & Livestock Commission, Milton Keynes.

MLC, (1982a) *Group Breeding Schemes for Sheep*. Meat & Livestock Commission, Milton Keynes.

MLC (1983) *Sheep Yearbook*. Meat & Livestock Commission, Milton Keynes.

MLC (1984) *Lamb Vaccination*. Meat & Livestock Commission, Milton Keynes.

MLC (1984a) *Sheep Yearbook*. Meat & Livestock Commission, Milton Keynes.

MLC (1984b) *Data Sheet 84/3*. Meat & Livestock Commission, Milton Keynes.

MLC (1988a) *Feeding the Ewe*. Meat & Livestock Commission, Milton Keynes.

MLC (1988b) *Sheep in Britain*. Meat & Livestock Commission, Milton Keynes.

MLC (1988c) *Data Sheet 88/3*. Meat & Livestock Commission, Milton Keynes.

MLC (1989) *Lamb Carcase Production*. Meat & Livestock Commission, Milton Keynes.

MLC (1989a) *Sheep Yearbook*. Meat & Livestock Commission, Milton Keynes.

MLC (1990) *Sheep Yearbook*. Meat & Livestock Commission, Milton Keynes.

MLC (1991) *Sheep Yearbook*. Meat & Livestock Commission, Milton Keynes.

MLC (1992a) *Sheep Yearbook*. Meat & Livestock Commission, Milton Keynes.

MLC (1992b) *UK Weekly* (series). Meat & Livestock Commission, Milton Keynes.

MLC (1992c) *International Meat Market Review*. Meat & Livestock Commission, Milton Keynes.

Nitter, G. (1978) Breed utilisation for meat production in sheep. *Animal Breeding Abstracts*, **46**, 131–43.

NSA (1992) *British Sheep*. National Sheep Association, Malvern.

Orr, R.J., Parsons, A.J., Treacher, T.T. & Penning, P.D. (1988) Seasonal patterns of grass production under cutting or continuous stocking managements. *Grass and Forage Science*, **43**, 199–208.

Parsons, A.J. (1984) Management guidelines for continuously grazed swards. *Grass Farmer* No. **17**, 5–9.

Penning, P.D., Parsons, A.J., Orr, R.J. & Treacher, T.T. (1991) Intake and behaviour responses by sheep to changes in sward characteristics under continuous stocking. *Grass and Forage Science*, **46**, 15–28.

Pollott, G.E. (1979) The development of lamb production systems using one type of Sudanese sheep. *World Review of Animal Production*, **15**, 57–68.

Pollott, G.E., Flamant, J.C., Jankowski, S., Tchakerian, E. & Trodahl, S. (1987) Report of the EAAP Sheep and Goat Commission working group on data collection schemes for the evaluation of production systems. *38th Annual Meeting of European Association for Animal Production*, Lisbon.

Pollott, G.E. & Kilkenny, J.B. (1976a) A note on the use of condition scoring in commercial sheep flocks. *Animal Production*, **23**, 261–4.

Pollott, G.E. & Kilkenny, J.B. (1976b) A scheme for grassland recording based on the livestock unit concept. *Animal Production*, **22**, 147 (abstract).

Ponting, K. (1980) *Sheep of the World*. Blandford Press Ltd, Poole.

Rhind, S.M. (1992) Nutrition: its effects on reproductive performance and its hormonal control in female sheep and goats. In: *Progress in Sheep and Goat Research*. (ed. A. Speedy). CAB International, Wallingford.

Robinson, J.J. (1990) Nutrition over the winter period – the breeding female. In: *New Developments in Sheep Production*. (eds C.F.R. Slade & T.L.J. Lawrence). British Society of Animal Production, Edinburgh.

Russel, A.J.F., Doney, J.M. & Gunn, R.G. (1969) Subjective assessment of body fat in live sheep. *Journal of Agricultural Science*, Cambridge, **72**, 451–4.

Rutter, W. (1983) Grassland management for the lowland ewe. In: *Sheep Production*. (ed. W. Haresign), pp. 207–18. Butterworths, London.

SAC (1992) *Farm Management Handbook*. Scottish Agricultural College, Edinburgh.

Simm, G. (1987) Carcass evaluation in sheep breeding programmes. In: *New Techniques in Sheep Production*. (eds. I.F.M. Marai & J.B. Owen). Butterworths, London.

Simm, G. (1992) Selection for lean meat production in sheep. In: *Progress in Sheep and Goat Research*. (ed. A. Speedy). CAB International, Wallingford.

Simm, G., Dingwall, W.S., Murphy, S.V. & Brown, W.R. (1990) Selection for improved carcass composition in terminal sire sheep breeds. In: *New Developments in Sheep Production*. (eds C.F.R. Slade & T.L.J. Lawrence). BSAP, Occasional Publication No. 14. British Society of Animal Production, Edinburgh.

Spedding, A. (1984) Alternative Enterprises. *Milk Marketing Board Conference*. MMB, Taunton.

Tempest, W.M. (1983) Management of the frequent lambing flock. In: *Sheep Production*. (ed. W. Haresign), pp. 467–82. Butterworths, London.

Thomas, C., Reeve, A. & Fisher, G.E.J. (1991) *Milk from Grass*. British Grassland Society, Reading.

Treacher, T.T. (1990) Grazing management and supplementation for the lowland sheep flock. In: *New Developments in Sheep Production*. (eds C.F.R. Slade & T.L.J. Lawrence). BSAP Occasional Publication No. 14. British Society of Animal Productions, Edinburgh.

Vipond, J.E., Swift, G., McClelland, T.H. & Milne, J.A. (1990) Evaluation of a perennial ryegrass and small-leaved clover sward without nitrogen fertilizer under continuous sheep grazing at a controlled sward height. In: *New Developments in Sheep Production*. (eds C.F.R. Slade & T.L.J. Lawrence). BSAP Occasional Publication No. 14. British Society of Animal Production, Edinburgh.

Weiner, G. (1979) Breed substitution and cross breeding as a means of increasing productivity. In: *The Management and Diseases of Sheep*. (ed. British Council.) British Council and Commonwealth Agricultural Bureau, London.

White, I.R. & Russel, A.J.F. (1987) Pregnancy diagnosis and foetal determination. In: *New Techniques in Sheep Production*. (eds I.F.M. Marai & J.B. Owen). Butterworths, London.

Wildig, J. (1980) The economics of the Pwllpeiran Mountain pasture improvement scheme. *BGS Occasional Symposium No. 12*. British Grassland Society, Reading.

Wildig, J., Richards, R.I.W.A. & Roberts, M. (1982) The effect of land improvement and better winter feeding on the physical and financial output of a mountain sheep farm. *Experimental Husbandry*, **38**, 138–53.

Index

Africa, 23, 30
agistment, 153
Agricultural Development and Advisory
    Service (ADAS), 9
Agricultural Training Boards (ATB), 133
Agrostis-Festuca, 162
Animal Breed Research Organization
    (ABRO), 79, 106
annual ewe premium, 41, 42
appetite, 69, 71
Araganese, 32
Argentina, 34, 44
artificial insemination, 75–6, 97
Asia, 19, 21, 22, 23, 30
Astrakhan, 31
Australia, 19, 22, 25, 26, 31, 44, 60, 99,
    105, 109, 141
Awassi, 32

barley, 68
barren ewes, 66
Belgium, 177
Berrichon du Cher, 97
Bluefaced Leicester, 78, 144, 164, 168,
    173
BLUP (Best Linear Unbiased
    Prediction), 95, 97, 100, 107
boneless cuts, 86
Border Leicester, 78, 144, 164, 168, 172
breed
    improvement, 95
    liveweight, 78, 80, 89, 90
    substitution, 58–60
breeding
    ewes, 55–72, 172, 184
    rams, 72–6, 180
    value, 95, 96, 100, 101
Beulah Speckleface, 107, 172

Cambridge, 106

CAMDA, 95, 106
capital, 35, 37, 133–6
    investment in hill flocks, 162
carcase
    assessment on live animal, 97–8
    characteristics, 77–83, 98
    classification, 78, 83–5, 90
    composition, 78, 79
    damage, 92–3
    production, 179
    weight, 48, 73, 83, 84, 86, 90, 91, 141,
        177, 184
cash flow, 134, 182
census data, 47
certification, 41
Charlollais, 107, 142, 187
cheese, 30
Chile, 43
clawback, 41
clean grazing, 14, 74
clover, 115–16, 157, 159
colostrum, 69
Columbia, 35, 141
concentrates, 64, 69, 74, 127–8
conception rate, 60, 76
condition scoring, 8, 60–64, 65, 67, 68,
        70, 71, 72, 74, 83, 166
conformation, 41, 73, 80, 83–5, 88, 97, 99
conservation, 122, 126–7
contemporary comparison, 96, 100, 101
Coopworth, 141
Cormo, 34
Corriedale, 34, 141
crossbred ewes, 57, 168, 172, 173
crossbreeding, 58–60, 143
    in Britain, 143
cull ewes, 49, 178–9
    survey, 179
Czechoslovakia, 43

D value, 127
Dalesbred, 167
Dohne Merino, 141
Dorset Down, 79, 80
Dorset Horn, 57, 58, 59, 180, 184
draft ewes, 49, 145, 155, 164, 166
dry matter of grass, 12, 112–13

early-lambing systems, 182–5
early weaning, 81, 96
East of Scotland College, 14, 96
EC, 2, 150
    Budgetary Stabilizer, 41
    Common Agricultural Policy (CAP),
        39
    production, 88
    sheepmeat regime, 28, 32, 39, 42, 134,
        151
England, 9, 110, 144–6, 168, 180
environmental effects, 99, 100
equipment, 139
Europe, 19, 25, 26, 32
European Currency Units (ECU), 43
ewe age, 99
    lambs, 67, 172
    replacements, 82–3
Exeter University, 9
extensive production, 34, 36

Farm Buildings Information Centre,
    138
fat class, 41, 78, 80–85, 92
feed blocks, 127, 157, 165
feedlots, 142
fertility, 56
ffrid, 156, 162
finished lambs, 176
Finnish Landrace, 58, 59, 143, 184
fishmeal, 69
fixed costs, 4, 129, 130
fleece quality, 99
fleeceweight, 99, 141
flock health, 15
flock replacement cost, 3, 176
Flockplan, 3, 5, 9, 152, 176, 178, 180
flushing, 65
foetal growth, 67, 69–70
foetal loss, 66
Food and Agriculture Organisation of
    the United Nations (FAO), 19
forage crops, 11, 124–6, 190
France, 30, 31, 32, 39, 56, 83, 96, 136,
    142, 146, 177, 179

generation interval, 102
genetic
    control, 102
    improvement, 93–108
    potential, 77
    progress, 101, 102, 104
genotype-environment interaction, 59
Germany, 44, 96, 177
Gotland, 31
grass, 5, 109–23
    costs, 189
    dry matter production, 111
    growing days, 110, 111
    growth, 112
    height, 118–20
    utilization, 116–17, 120–21
    varieties, 115
grassland, 151
    costs, 121, 122
    improvement, 157
    in Britain, 110–11
    management, 189
    recording, 122–3
    site class, 114, 117
    use, 5, 11
grazing systems, 116–17, 157
Great Britain, 109, 143, 149, 177, 179
Greece, 44
Greenland, 43
Greyface, 164, 167, 172, 191
gross margin, 3–4
groundnut, 69
group breeding schemes, 97, 105–107
growth rate, 77, 79
guide prices, 41

Hampshire Down, 35, 78, 79, 80, 188,
    198
hay, 65–73, 127
hefts, 156
heritability, 98, 99, 102
Hill Cheviot, 167
hill ewe population, 151–3
Hill Farming Research Organisation
    (HFRO), 60, 155, 158
hill flocks, 141, 151
    output, 156–61
    pastures, 151
    resources, 153–6
    results, 152–6
Holland, 141
housing, 136–40
Hungary, 44

hybrid vigour, 60, 146
hypothermia, 82

Ile de France, 59, 78, 96, 136
import quotas, 43
inbreeding, 103
India, 22
indoor finishing of hill lambs, 161
industry data, 9
intervention, 41
investment capital, 135–6, 159
Ireland, 39, 80
Italy, 44, 142

Japan, 26

Karakul, 31

labour, 132–3
  costs, 129
Lacaune, 30, 56
lactation, 70–72
lamb
  cutting, 28, 29, 30
  growth, 60, 71, 77–83, 96, 97, 99, 100, 105
  handling points, 90–92
  sales, 56, 74, 176
  selection, 88
  survival, 35, 56, 60, 70, 82
  value, 5
lambing percentage, 61
land, 131–2
  improvement, 156
lean percentage, 79, 98
Less Favoured Areas Directive, 150, 151, 166
LI (Lean Index), 104
lime, 157
Liscombe EHF, 160
litter size, 56, 99, 102, 104
livestock units, 123
Lleyn, 107, 180
lowland systems, 180–96
  early lambing, 180–85
  grass and forage, 189–92
  grass finishing, 185–9
  store lamb finishing, 193–6

maize, 69
Manchega, 32, 142
market requirements, 85–7, 177
market support, 41

marketing, 83–93
Masham, 164, 167
maternal characters, 56–8
maternal performance, 60
mating, 62, 66
mature size, 57, 99, 104
Meat and Livestock Commission (MLC), 3, 5, 28, 47, 129, 145, 154, 155, 166, 168, 169, 186
Mediterranean, 142
Merino, 25, 32, 34, 36, 141, 142
Middle East, 23, 26, 27, 142
milk-fed lambs, 180
milk production, 23, 56, 70, 71, 82, 99, 142
Ministry of Agriculture, Fisheries and Food (MAFF), 14, 154
Molina caerulea, 157, 159
mothering ability, 56
Mule, 59, 167–8

National Sheep Association (NSA), 47
net margin, 4, 130
New Zealand, 19, 25, 30, 31, 43, 44, 99, 105, 132, 141
nitrogen, 113–14, 174
North County Cheviot, 26, 78, 79, 167
Norway, 3, 29, 33, 96–7, 104
nucleus flock, 95, 105–107
nutrition
  of ewes, 10, 11, 64–72, 83
  of lambs, 81–2

oats, 68
Oceania, 19, 21
oestrus synchronization, 60, 76
on-farm testing, 98
out-of-season breeding, 57
ovulation rate, 56, 62, 66, 166
Oxford Down, 59, 78, 79

Pacific Islands, 19
Patagonia, 34
performance records, 8–10, 73, 94, 100, 176
performance testing, 95–6
planning, 1
  aids, 6–10
Poland, 44
Poll Dorset, 57, 180, 184
predators, 35
pregnancy
  scanning, 69, 179

toxemia, 68, 70
pregnant mare's serum gonadotrophin
    (PMSG), 60, 76
products, 22–31
    upland, 166–8
    lowland, 176–80
progeny testing, 96–7, 105
progesterone, 60
protein
    degradation, 69, 71
    requirement, 69, 71, 81
purebreeding, 140–41
Pwllpeiran EHF, 135, 154, 162

raddle, 74
raking, 156
Rambouillet, 35
ram
    circles, 96, 104
    management, 74
    selection, 73
Rare Breeds Survival Trust, 180
rationing, 65
Redesdale EHF, 156, 159, 160, 165
reseeding, 158, 165
Romanov, 31, 59, 97, 143, 146
Romney, 25, 107, 143

saleable yield, 28, 29, 86
Scotland, 9, 28, 29, 110, 146, 152, 156,
    167, 172
Scottish Agricultural Colleges, 9, 96, 130
Scottish Blackface, 141, 143, 154, 155,
    165, 167, 172
Scottish Halfbred, 164, 167, 168, 189
selection
    criterion, 33, 99, 101
    index, 33, 94, 95, 100, 101
    intensity, 101, 102
    objective, 94–5, 101, 105
semen scoring, 75
Sheepbreeder scheme, 99
sheep products, 23–31
    hair, 37
    meat, 26, 27, 28, 29, 34, 35, 37, 39, 44
    milk, 30, 39
    skins, 23, 31, 39
    wool, 23, 25, 26, 27, 39
silage 127
Sire referencing schemes, 107
South Africa, 141
South America, 19, 21, 109, 141
Southdown, 79, 80

soyabean meal, 69, 70
Spain, 32, 59, 132, 136, 142
SQQ (standard quality quotation), 49
stocking rate, 5, 64, 117, 174, 186
store lamb, 12–13, 49, 156, 166, 178, 193
    fattening, 156
straw, 127
subcutaneous fat, 79, 84–6
subsidy, 150
Sudan, 36
Suffolk, 35, 59, 79, 80, 96, 107, 164, 171,
    172, 180, 184, 188, 189, 192
Swaledale, 141, 143, 154, 167, 173
Syria, 142
systematic crossbreeding, 60, 143–8

tack, 153
targets, 5, 171, 174
Teeswater, 164, 167
terminal sire, 74, 78, 97, 98, 100, 107, 143,
    145, 147
Texel, 78, 79, 80, 96, 107, 141
threshold flock, 41
top third, 5, 57, 120
    hill, 155
    lowland, 183, 187
    upland, 169–70
trade, 44
transhumance, 32
Turkey, 22
twin splitting, 160
two-pasture system, 157–8

UK
    ewe population, 19, 38, 46, 47, 164, 175
    market price, 49
    production, 46
    slaughterings, 48
ultrasonic scanning, 68, 70, 98, 107, 162,
    179
utilized metabolisable energy (UME),
    123
USA, 35, 109, 136, 142
USSR, 19, 21, 23, 25, 26, 31, 36

vaccination, 31, 73, 74, 93
variable costs, 4
variable premium, 41
    scheme, 41
Voluntary Restraint Agreement, 43, 44

Wales, 9, 107, 110, 145, 151, 156, 162,
    167, 168, 172

weaning, 66, 81, 154
weight, 8
  eight-week, 99, 100
Welsh Halfbred, 160, 167
Welsh Mountain, 27, 95, 106, 141, 143,
  154, 164, 165, 167, 172
Welsh Mule, 164, 167
Wensleydale, 78, 79
wheat, 69
within-breed variation, 57, 58

within-flock selection, 104, 105, 141
wool, 8, 58, 74, 142, 166, 176, 178
Wool Marketing Board, 138, 178
working capital, 133–5
world sheep population, 19–22
world trade, 22
Wrzosowka, 31

X-ray computed tomography, 98